Artsy Fartsy

Cultural History of the Fart

Volume Two

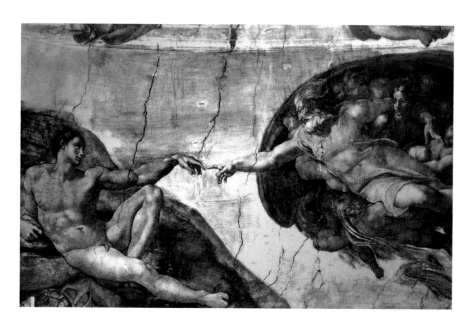

Joseph B. Weiss, MD, FACP, FACG, AGAF
Clinical Professor of Medicine,
Gastroenterology
University of California, San Diego

Copyright © 2016 Joseph B. Weiss, MD
        SmartAsk Books
        Rancho Santa Fe, California, USA
        www.smartaskbooks.com

ISBN-13: 978-1-943760-17-6 Volume Two Color
ISBN-13: 978-1-943760-40-4 Volume Two B&W
ISBN-13: 978-1-943760-35-0 Volume Two e-Book Color
ISBN-13: 978-1-943760-03-9 Combined Volumes Color

Last digit is the print number: 9 8 7 6 5 4 3

Dedication

This volume is dedicated to clearing the air of the misperception that a fart is anything other than a normal physiologic process common to all humanity. Nature and natural processes should be universally accepted as one of the cherished principles of basic human rights.

I am indebted to my loved ones, Nancy, Danielle, Jeremy, Courie, Lizzy & Indy who have offered their insights, suggestions, comments, and unwavering support throughout the long process of having this project finally come to pass. You will always be the mighty wind beneath my wings.

I. **Table of Contents**

II. **Preface**   VIII

III. **Introduction**   1

IV. **Etymology - Origin of the Word Fart**   4

V. **Physiology - Digestion and the Fart**   7

VI. **Chronology of Fart in the Arts (Volume One)**

   Hieronymus Bosch
   Michelangelo di Lodovico Buonarroti Simoni
   Pieter Bruegel the Elder
   Medieval Manuscripts
   Francisco Goya
   Wolfgang Amadeus Mozart
   James Gillray
   Louis-Léopold Boilly
   Richard Newton
   Japanese Lithographs Edo Period
   Utagawa Kuniyoshi
   George Cruikshank
   S. Stoutshanks
   Richard Wagner
   Aubrey Beardsley
   Joseph Pujol (Le Pétomane)
   James Ensor
   Canadian Broadcast Corporation
   Salvador Dali
   Cinematic Arts
   Bollywood Hindi Movies
   Seinfeld
   Mr. Methane
   Budweiser Super Bowl Commercial
   The Lion King
   Cartoonists
   Children's Book Art
   The Simpsons
   Family Guy
   South Park
   Beavis & Butt-Head
   Chen Wenlin
   Ontario Ministry of Health
   Advertising & Marketing

VII. Chronology of Fart in History (Volume One)

Bel-Phegor
Bible Prophets
Pythagoras
Herodotus
Hippocrates
Aristotle
Metrocles
Cicero
Claudius
Seneca
Flavius Josephus
Plutarch
Babylonian Talmud
Elagabalus
Whoopee Cushion
Yoga
St. Jerome
Augustine of Hippo (St. Augustine)
Islam Hadith
Sir Thomas Moore
Desiderius Erasmus
Martin Luther
HRH Queen Elizabeth I
Michel de Montaigne
Henry Ludlow
Oliver Cromwell
Lord John Wilmot, Earl of Rochester
Benjamin Franklin
Thomas Blount
Immanuel Kant
Charles James Fox
Abraham Lincoln
Sir Richard Burton
John Gregory Bourke
Sigmund Freud
T.E. Lawrence of Arabia
Sir Winston Churchill
Adolf Hitler
Josef Stalin
Sir Robert Hutchinson
Charles de Gaulle
Lyndon Baines Johnson
Ronald Reagan
H.M. Queen Elizabeth II
George W. Bush

Muammar Gaddafi
H.H. the 14th Dalai Lama of Tibet
Global Warming

VIII. Chronology of Fart in Literature (Volume Two)   **21**
Bel-Phegor
Aristophanes
Petronius
Marcus Valerius Martialis
Arabian Nights
Dante Alighieri
Rutebeuf
William Langland
Geoffrey Chaucer
François Rabelais
John Heywood
William Shakespeare
Francois Béroalde de Verville
Ben Jonson
John Donne
Sir John Suckling
John Milton
John Aubrey
Daniel Defoe
Lord John Wilmot Earl of Rochester
Jonathon Swift
Voltaire
Henry Fielding
Jean Anthelme Brillat-Savarin
William Blake
Johann Wolfgang Von Goethe
Jacques Collin de Plancy
Honoré de Balzac
Victor Hugo
Edward Lear
Charles Pierre Baudelaire
Gustave Flaubert
Sir Richard Burton
Samuel Clemens (Mark Twain)
Émile Zola
James Joyce
D. H. Lawrence
Aldous Huxley
Henry Miller
Ernest Hemingway
Thomas Wolfe
W.H. Auden

Roald Dahl
Samuel Beckett
J.D. Salinger
Kurt Vonnegut, Jr.
Norman Mailer
William Styron
George MacDonald Fraser
John Barth
John Kennedy Toole
Philip Roth
George Carlin
Sir Salman Rushdie
James Patterson
Iain Banks
Howard Stern
Melina Marchetta
Children's Books

IX.   **Colloquialism, Idiom, & Synonym of Fart**   **140**

X.   **Fart in Foreign Languages**   **152**

XI.   **Afterword**   **155**

XII. **Index**   **159**

II. Preface

The book provides an entertaining overview of the fart in human culture and history, not an extensively referenced academic treatise. I expect that many will be surprised that the fart was a subject near to the hearts and minds of many illustrious and enlightened notables over the course of thousands of years of human history. The cultural mores of Western society have evolved and the fart has become a normal physiological event that has become more tolerated, although not yet universally accepted. Although the fart in human history has more than enough cultural value, I included some of the wisdom and maxims of the notables quoted to further enlighten the reader. It is my hope that *Artsy Fartsy, Cultural History of the Fart* is not only an informative and entertaining volume, but that the included content on digestion enhances the health and wellness of the reader. Hopefully, the reader will be stimulated to learn about their health and wellness in general, and about the digestive process in particular, as they read the subsequent entry on the origins of fart.

What is a fart, but a puff of nothingness, a wind of air? It is a weight so slight as to be immeasurable, a volume that can be compressed to fit on a pinhead. It can escape detection by stealth and silence, with odor so subtle as to be undetectable. It can give joyous pleasure and comfort to the one who releases it, and offence hostility, or amusement in others if detected. Of course, it can also grow in volume and intensity of sound and odor to magnify its presence to the point of being overwhelming. Even the word itself is a party to this paradox. How many words that describe a wind that can be so subtle and innocuous, find them banned from public discourse. The censorship of the word has played a role in modifying our literary heritage. Perhaps the passage in Shakespeare's *Romeo and Juliet*: "What's in a name? That which we call a rose, by any other name, would smell as sweet." was originally submitted as: "What's in a name? That which we call a fart, by any other name, would smell as tart." This volume is an anthology of human culture from the perspective of a small wind of nothingness. From nothing, the story of the fart in human culture magically expands its sphere of influence to virtually everything. Art, literature, music, science, medicine, cuisine, language, psychology, sociology, philosophy, humor, politics, are just a few of the disciplines that have been influenced by the fart. It has influenced individuals and society, from tyrants to saints, royalty to peasants, polymaths to fools.

In addition to providing an in depth overview of the fart in human culture, this volume also offers a selection of the non-fart wisdom and insights of the cultural illuminati who have contributed to the fart in the arts. The reader will hopefully enjoy and benefit from learning a great deal more about the nothingness of the fart, and the wisdom and culture of something more. As an author of a work of nonfiction, the primary purpose is to inform, educate, and entertain. On another level, the volume is also an allegorical tale about the limits imposed by culture and society on matters that arise in the world of nature outside of human control. It should come as no surprise that some of our greatest cultural works were considered both the apogee and zenith of the arts, with only the judgment of the times in which they were viewed discriminating between condemnation and accolades.

Many historical figures of note were branded heretics, tortured, and martyred only to be canonized and acclaimed saints and genius in later ages. The reverse is also true where celebrated leaders and thinkers have been exposed as charlatans and tyrants. So it best to suspend judgment and let the facts speak for themselves. Determine for yourself whether the fart is innocent and to be freely released, or is guilty and should be confined to the purgatory of the bowels of history.

III. Introduction

Artsy Fartsy, Cultural History of the Fart is a fascinating and factually correct review of the common fart through human culture and history. The cough, sneeze, hiccup, stomach rumble, burp, belch, and other bodily sounds simply cannot compete with the notoriety of the fart. Whether encountered live and in person or through the medium of literature, television, film, art, or music it may leave a powerful and lingering memory. The intent of this volume is to demonstrate that the ubiquitous fart has a more illustrious story to share than just lowbrow humor. The societal standards and cultural acceptance of this normal physiologic event have evolved over the years, and it is currently popular as a point of humor even in sophisticated circles.

To 'Air' is Human, Everything You Ever Wanted to Know About Intestinal Gas covers everything you ever wanted to know about the burp, belch, bloat, fart and everything digestive, but were either too afraid or too embarrassed to ask. Intestinal gas has been produced and released by virtually every human who has ever lived, yet very few people have been provided with the knowledge that can offer comfort and relief. This volume is overflowing with practical information, fascinating facts, surprising trivia, and tasteful humorous insight about this universal phenomenon.

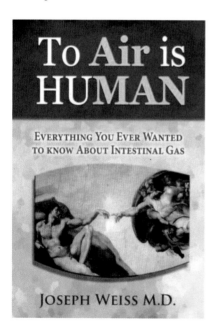

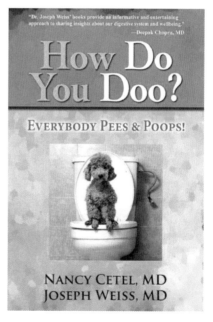

How Do You Doo? Everybody Pees & Poops! A delightfully informative, entertaining, and colorfully illustrated volume with valuable practical insights on toilet training. Tasteful color photographs of animals answering the call of nature allows the child to understand that everybody does it! Additional informative relevant content to entertain the adult while the child is 'on the potty' is included.

The Scoop on Poop! Flush with Knowledge is a uniquely informative tastefully entertaining, and well-illustrated volume that is full of it! The 'it' being a comprehensive and knowledgeable overview of all topics related to the remains of the digestive process. Whether you call it poop, feces, excrement, manure, dung, or the hundred plus other euphemisms, shit happens, and it happens a lot! Tens of billions of pounds and kilograms of it or deposited every day by while diversity of animal and microbial life. Humans alone contribute over three billion pounds a day, and only a small percentage of that is treated by a sewage system

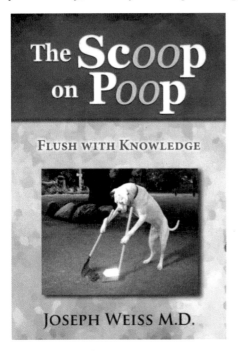
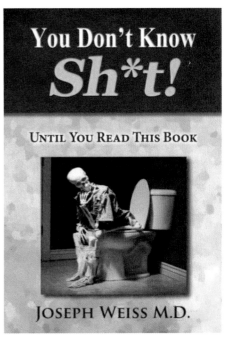

The identical content of The Scoop on Poop has been provocatively and cheekily retitled as *You Don't Know Sh*t! Until You Read This Book*. This volume is an informative, entertaining and colorfully illustrated fountain of knowledge that is full of valuable information, including eccentricities and peculiarities, about the remains of the digestive process. Although this end result is politely described as feces or excrement, it is more commonly known by one of oldest words in the English language, shit. The book covers everything you ever wanted to know about this subject. Whether you disdain it, or appreciate it, it is part of the human (and animal) experience. The purpose of this volume is to share rarely discussed but very important knowledge about poop. The information ranges from the potentially life-saving to the sidesplitting descriptions of the eccentricities and peculiarities of human behavior on the subject matter. The wealth of information and trivia can sustain a long social conversation, or cut it short abruptly!

AirVeda: Ancient & New Medical Wisdom, Digestion & Gas covers the remarkable advances in the understanding of digestive health and wellness. New information about the critical role of genomics, epigenetics, the gut microbiome, and the gut-brain-microbiome-diet axis are opening new avenues to optimal whole body health and wellness. An appreciation of the ancient wisdom of Ayurveda and other disciplines shows that they had advanced insights into the nature of the human body and the holistic approach. Although intestinal gas, basic bodily functions, and feces have been topics culturally suppressed, knowledge and understanding are needed to achieve and maintain optimal health. This volume, and others in the series, provide an informative and entertaining in depth look at the amazing world of human health and digestion.

"Ayurveda is a 5,000 year old system of natural healing that reminds us that health is the balanced and dynamic integration between our environment, body, mind and spirit. In Dr. Joseph Weiss' book, AirVeda, he provides an informative and entertaining approach to sharing insights about our digestive system and wellbeing by applying the ancient wisdom of Ayurveda to everyday life." **Deepak Chopra, MD**

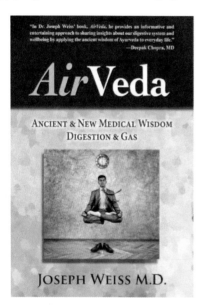

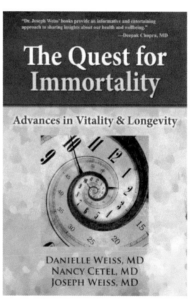

The Quest for Immortality, Advances in Vitality & Longevity provides an informative and enlightening overview of the remarkable advances in science and medicine that are dramatically enhancing human health and lifespan. The volume is written in clear, understandable, and engaging language with striking colorful illustrations. From groundbreaking nanotechnology to genomics and stem cells, the secrets of vitality and longevity are being uncovered along with more traditional advances and practical insights into disease prevention and health enhancement. The website www.smartaskbooks.com has a complete listing of books and programs by Joseph Weiss, MD, FACP, FACG, AGAF, Clinical Professor of Medicine (Gastroenterology), University of California, San Diego.

IV Etymology - Origin of the Word Fart

English is the richest language on the planet, with more words by far than any other. This is due to the significant influence of its history of foreign invasion and occupation, especially during the days of the Roman Empire. Unlike other conquerors, the Romans did not impose the Latin language on the inhabitants of the British Isles. The population adapted their own native tongue to include words borrowed from occupiers and foreign influences to rapidly expand the English vocabulary.

The word fart is the correct word to use in the English language, and indeed is one of its oldest words. The alternative words used, such as flatus and flatulence are not originally English words as they have been borrowed from the Latin, where their general meaning is of a wind or a blowing.

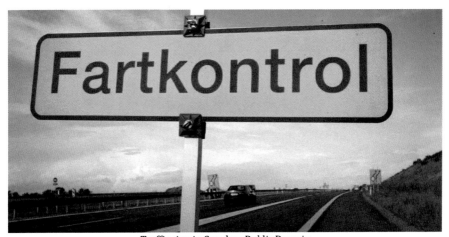
Traffic sign in Sweden, Public Domain

There is controversy as to the derivation of the word fart. It is thought to have Indo-European roots in the Germanic language word farzen. The word fart may have originated as onomatopoeia, a word that phonetically imitates the sound of the event it describes. Another thought is that it was related to the term for partridge, as the bird makes a similar sound when it is disturbed in its natural habitat and takes flight. How it made that transition may be an enlightening example of the evolution of words and language.

The Indo-European word *perd* means fart, and this led to the Latin word *pedere* meaning the verb to fart, and *peditum* the noun fart. The Indo-European *perd* led to the Greek word for fart πέρδομαι *perdomai*. It is also cognate with Sanskrit *pardate*, Avestan *pərəδaiti*, Italian *fare un peto*, French "péter", Russian пердеть (perdet') and Polish "pierd".

The related Greek word *perdix* referred to a type of bird that made an explosive fart like sound when it was flushed from the brush when startled. While being incorporated from Greek to Old French it became *perdriz*, then Middle English *partrich*, and finally Modern English *partridge*. The final step would be to complete the circuitous history and modify it to the name *fartridge*!

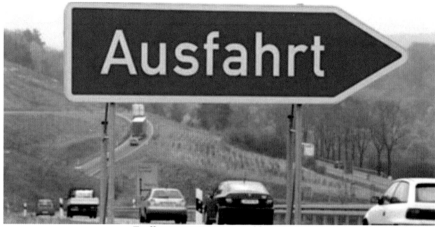

Traffic sign in Germany, Public Domain

The word fart is also found in other languages, but there it often has a different and unrelated meaning. In the Scandinavian languages it usually denotes speed or motion. In Danish and Norwegian it is often used in combination with other words that obscures the meaning even more. For example in Danish a *fartcertifikate* means a trade certificate.

In Norwegian a *fart plan* means a schedule. The Norwegian phrase *stå på fartin* pronounced as stop-a–fartin means ready to leave. Likewise the phrase *farts måler* pronounced as fart smeller refers to a speedometer. In Swedish a speed bump is called a *farthinder*. *Fartlek* is speed training by running at alternate intervals of fast and slow paces.

Likewise if you travel on a Scandinavian marine vessel you may see the control of engine speed labeled as *half fart* and *full fart* for half speed and full speed respectively. Fart kontrol zones are speed zones. In Germany a similar word *fahrt* means a journey, trip, tour, or passage. It is often seen in signs that say e*infahrt* (sounds like in-fart) and *ausfahrt* (sounds like out-fart) denoting entrance and exit respectively.

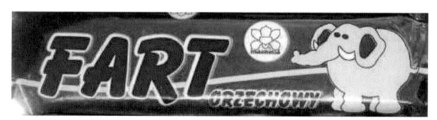

In Spanish and Portuguese *fart* means an excess of anything, especially a food. One of the richest deserts they offer is called a *farte*, which means a fruit tarte in Spain and usually a sugar almond or cream cake in Portugal. In Italy the word *farto* means mattress. In Hungarian *fartaj* means buttocks. In Poland if you want to buy a popular candy bar with a name that means lucky you will be looking for a *Fart* bar.

Several languages have a number of different words for variations of a theme for which there is only one word in English. The word snow is one example where we have a singular word, but the Inuit, Eskimo, Aleut, Sami and other languages of the native people of the Arctic and northern latitudes may have hundreds of words.

When it comes to the word fart, the English language is very limited with just the singular word. I will not leap to the conclusion that the language that has the most words for fart needed to do so for necessity. Their population may or may not have the world's highest rate of fart production, but they certainly have the most descriptive fart words.

The Russian words for fart include *perdyozh* (first act of breaking wind), *perdun* (perpetrator and outcome), *perdil'nik* (place from where it comes), *Perun* (ancient God of wind), *bzdun* (silent fart), *bzdyukha* (silent fart as well as a stupid jerk). Some of the Russian verbs for the action of farting are particularly colorful. *Perdet'* (to fart with or without sound), *bzdet'* (to fart silently), *pereperdet* (to fart repeatedly), and my favorite word *nabzdet'sya* (to fart silently to one's complete and utter satisfaction!).

V. Physiology – Digestion and the Fart

Farts are ubiquitous, all living creatures generate gas from the cellular respiration of metabolism, and humans are no exception. The bacteria in your colonic flora generate microscopic nanofarts and microfarts, which collect into larger bubbles of gas in the bowel. They are intermixed with the atmospheric air swallowed throughout the day and particularly at meals.

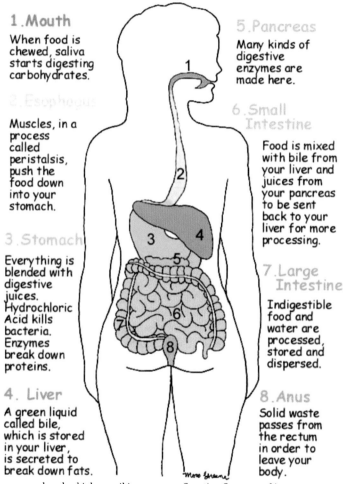

1.Mouth
When food is chewed, saliva starts digesting carbohydrates.

2.Esophagus
Muscles, in a process called peristalsis, push the food down into your stomach.

3.Stomach
Everything is blended with digestive juices. Hydrochloric Acid kills bacteria. Enzymes break down proteins.

4. Liver
A green liquid called bile, which is stored in your liver, is secreted to break down fats.

5.Pancreas
Many kinds of digestive enzymes are made here.

6.Small Intestine
Food is mixed with bile from your liver and juices from your pancreas to be sent back to your liver for more processing.

7.Large Intestine
Indigestible food and water are processed, stored and dispersed.

8.Anus
Solid waste passes from the rectum in order to leave your body.

hawkesbiology.wikispaces.com Creative Commons License

Aerophagia is universal and we swallow on average three to five milliliters (one teaspoonful) of air with every swallow. Even when we are not eating or drinking we regularly swallow the saliva we produce. The average human swallows over two thousand times a day. Chewing gum, hard candies, and use of chewing or smoking tobacco or other recreational products increase the volume of air swallowed. Drinking through a straw, directly from a can or bottle, or talking while eating, will also increase the amount of air swallowed. Ill-fitting dentures may also contribute to aerophagia. Another common source of swallowed air is contained within the foods we eat. An apple is forty percent air by volume, and bread is over sixty percent air by volume. If you compress an apple or a loaf of bread you will see that they a sizeable portion of their total volume is air. Whipped foods, soufflés, and baked goods, all have high air content.

Have you ever forgotten to put an ice cream container back in the freezer. Ice cream is typically forty percent air by volume and when it melts the air escapes and the full container is no longer full. By the way, the ice cream industry knows that adding air, known in the as overage, enhances the mouth feel texture of the ice cream and adds forty percent to the profit margin because ice cream is sold by volume, not by weight. Besides the swallowed air, additional gasses are produced during the enzymatic digestive processes, as well as the neutralization of gastric hydrochloric acid and pancreatic and duodenal bicarbonate. The end result is that a large volume of gasses transit the bowel and may be eliminated as a fart. Fortunately the vast majority of the gasses produced are absorbed by the gut and then into the bloodstream through diffusion into a solution. The gasses leave the bloodstream when they arrive at the alveoli of the lungs where they are exhaled. The chemical component gasses have very different properties of diffusion through the bowel wall and into the bloodstream.

Carbon dioxide readily diffuses and enters solution and is readily exhaled. It is the largest component of the volume of gas generated in the proximal intestinal tract. It is a major contributor to the temporary distention and discomfort that commonly occurs after a meal. Carbonation is also utilized as a common beverage enhancer and adds to the volume of carbon dioxide gas in the stomach. Carbon dioxide is the most rapidly absorbed component of intestinal gas and is the easiest to eliminate by simply exhaling it in the breath. As very little remains in the bowel, it is only a minor component of a fart.

The volume of gasses in the gastrointestinal tract is dependent on many factors. This includes the quantity and nature of foods ingested and the body's ability to synthesize and utilize specific enzymes for the various food types. The nature and quantity of the bacteria in the gut flora influences the nature of intestinal gas both by their own active metabolism and by their ability to aid or hinder the digestive enzymes and processes.

One of the most common causes of excess gaseousness is deficiency of the enzyme lactase. Lactase hydrolyses the complex disaccharide dairy sugar lactose into the readily absorbable monosaccharide sugars glucose and galactose. With insufficient lactase the sugar molecule is not metabolized by the digestive system but is instead metabolized by the gut flora, also known as the microbiome. This results in gas production, and may also give rise to cramps and diarrhea.

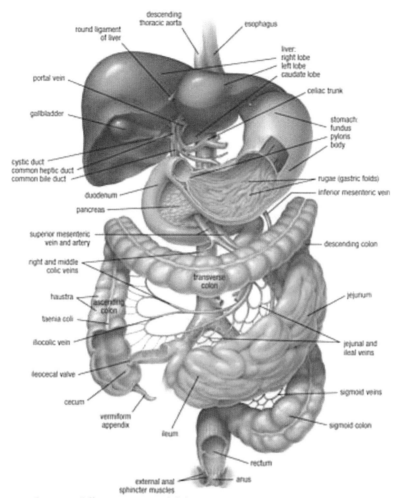

descending
thoracic aorta
round ligament
of liver
esophagus
liver:
right lobe
left lobe
caudate lobe
portal vein
celiac trunk
gallbladder
stomach:
fundus
pylorus
body
cystic duct
common hepatic duct
common bile duct
rugae (gastric folds)
inferior mesenteric vein
duodenum
pancreas
superior mesenteric
vein and artery
descending colon
right and middle
colic veins
transverse
colon
jejunum
haustra
ascending
colon
taenia coli
ileocolic vein
jejunal and
ileal veins
ileocecal valve
sigmoid veins
cecum
vermiform
appendix
sigmoid colon
ileum
rectum
external anal
sphincter muscles
anus

Openstax College courses.candelalearning.com Creative Commons License

Another food sugar that can cause excess gaseousness is commonly seen in fruit and is thus known as fructose. The human digestive system can handle a limited quantity of fructose at a time, and if the fruit intake exceeds this capacity the gut flora ferment this sugar with the release of gas, and often cramps and diarrhea.

That the microbes within our digestive tracts ferment foods that we have not fully digested is actually to our advantage, which is why the microbiome is considered essential to our good health. We can absorb some of the nutrients the microbes release in the fermentation process, including vitamins and bioactive molecules. We even use microbe fermentation in the preparation of many foods. When you add yeast to flour and watch the dough rise you are seeing the release of gasses from the fermentation process. The spongy character of bread and cakes, and why they are sixty percent air, is the result of gas production of the yeast fungus. The characteristic holes in Swiss cheese are the result of microbial gas production.

The entire production of wines, beer, and other alcohol beverages are based on microbial fermentation. In a parallel universe, we are actually ingesting the waste product of microbial fermentation.

Before you believe that a delicious baked good dependent on yeast farts loses some of its culinary appeal, please read on. A French pastry delicacy known as Pets de Nonne, also called **Pets de Sœurs**, is accurately translated as Nun's farts. These delicacies are a dessert puff pastry dating from medieval times and made from butter, milk, flour, sugar, eggs and sometimes honey is added. They are traditionally pan fried in lard and then baked. Their lightness inspired their name in French, Pets de Nonne and **Pets de Sœurs**. Another baked good named for its association with the fart is Pumpernickel (German: Devil's Fart) bread. It is a heavy dark brown bread traditionally made with coarsely ground rye flour and whole rye berries. It has been long associated with the Westphalia region of Germany for over 500 years. Like most rye breads it is traditionally made with an acidic sourdough starter, which inhibits the rye amylase enzymes. The name is associated with the coarse bread giving rise to flatulence.

Beans are known as the musical fruit because of the gas they produce in all humans. The reason for this is that legumes contain complex sugars known as raffinose, verbascose, and stachyose. Humans and other animals lack the enzyme, called alpha galactosidase, needed to metabolize these complex sugars into absorbable simple sugars. Without the enzyme the complex sugars are fermented by the gut microbiome producing gas. Aplha galactosidase is now commercially available as a dietary enzyme supplement to reduce the gas production associated with specific foods such as legumes.

Another enzyme that humans do not posses is cellulase, without which we cannot digest the cellulose found in most plants and grasses. Herbivorous animals do have those enzymes, which is why they can subsist on grazing of grasses and forage. Ruminant animals also heavily rely on the metabolic activity of the gut flora. The large volumes of gasses formed in their multi-chambered stomach are believed to be more significant contributors to global warming than their flatulence. Another factor in gas production is the speed of gastrointestinal transit. Drugs, hormones, food products, and illness may influence this. The absorptive capacity and health of the mucosal lining, and the physical length of the individual's gastrointestinal tract also play a role. The often-quoted figure of twelve farts per day is a reasonable approximation of the average number of farts passed, but there is a very wide range of what is considered normal.

Besides the numerical quantity of farts passed per day is the question of what is considered a normal volume of gas passed. If you are familiar with physics, a series of natural laws were defined that express the relationship between temperature, pressure, and volume. The relationship between temperature and pressure is direct, i.e. the higher the temperature, the larger the volume of space a given number of molecules a gas would occupy. The expansion to a larger volume of occupied space may result in intestinal bloating, discomfort, and increased burping and farting. The relationship with pressure is indirect, i.e. the greater the pressure the smaller the volume.

We would rarely experience a change in intestinal gas volume based on temperature. On the contrary, we will often experience significant changes in volume due to pressure. Increases in pressure reduce the volume of gas, which is not a problem when it comes to the gut and our symptoms of gas. It can become a major problem when the pressure decreases and the gas volume increases. The atmospheric pressure changes rapidly as we go higher or lower from sea level. The effects on intestinal gas are seen in scuba divers, pilots, airplane passengers, mountain climbers, living at higher elevations, and even taking an elevator to the top of a skyscraper. When the pressure change is rapid, for example a scuba diver returning to the surface, or an astronaut on ascent to orbit, the consequences can be dramatic and life threatening and are known as barotrauma.

Most gasses that are commercially available (oxygen, helium, air, etc.) are compressed and contained in hardened metal canisters that can withstand very high pressure. This allows for significant savings of space, for example allowing scuba divers to have the equivalent of a roomful of air within a single tank. The intestinal tract is flexible and expandable to a degree, more like a balloon than a metal container. As such changes in the surrounding atmospheric pressure can result in large volume changes, which in the extreme of barotrauma may lead to perforation and rupture.

Chemical Composition of Flatulence

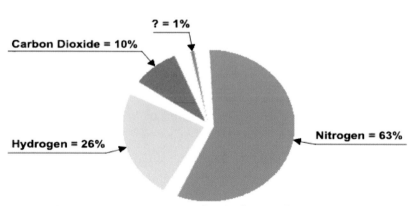

www.pyroenergen.com Creative Commons License

The fart would not be as notorious as it is if it were not for its aroma. Over ninety - nine percent of the gasses in a fart are odorless. While a number of individuals may have methane present in their farts, methane is odorless. If you smell a natural gas (methane) leak it is not the methane you smell, but an odorant gas added by the gas company as a safety precaution to give notice of danger.

The majority of the aroma from a fart comes from hydrogen sulfide, skatole, indole, and aromatic fatty acids, the majority coming from the digestion of animal fats. While vegetarians may fart more than carnivores, the aroma is not nearly as pungent or offensive. For those interested in a more in-depth account of the fascinating natural history of intestinal gas (and its consequences of burping, bloating, and farting), the volume *To 'Air' is Human* is an enjoyable and definitive resource. In the meanwhile, before delving into the cultural history of the fart, a brief overview of digestion would be appropriate.

All of the attention on the physiologic origin of farts makes it sound like the primary purpose of the digestive tract is their creation for your annoyance or amusement. Of course, the purpose of the digestive tract is to support life by providing the nutrition and energy we need for all of our body functions. Intestinal gas is simply a natural waste product, and is rarely of consequence. As such, in my humble yet expert opinion, it should be utilized as a source of amusement or cultural enlightenment.

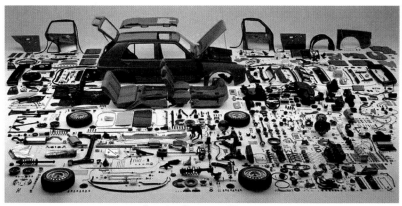

Creative Commons License

Perhaps the analogy is not the best one, but think of the digestive tract as the reverse of the assembly line, a disassembly line. A factory has a goal to be efficient and profitable, and may not win too many awards for architecture and beauty. So too with the digestive tract, the process has been refined over eons of evolution, yet still have its primitive origins and end products.

We begin our factory tour with a view much like you would get sitting in your car going through a car wash. Before you even go to the car wash, your brain has to make the conscious decision that this activity is what it wants to do. In the same manner, the brain begins the digestive process with the decision to satisfy its hunger call, or because an appetizing opportunity presents itself. When thinking about food and eating, the brain may activate the secretion of saliva and prime the digestive processes of the stomach and internal organs.

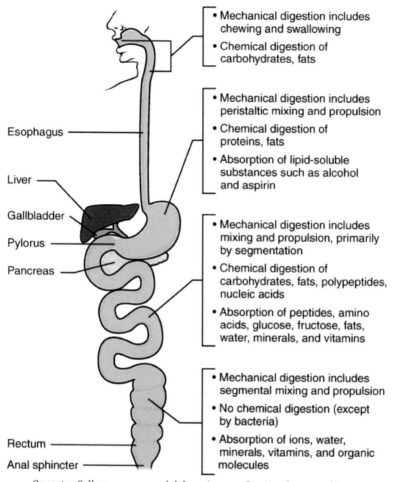

- Mechanical digestion includes chewing and swallowing
- Chemical digestion of carbohydrates, fats

- Mechanical digestion includes peristaltic mixing and propulsion
- Chemical digestion of proteins, fats
- Absorption of lipid-soluble substances such as alcohol and aspirin

- Mechanical digestion includes mixing and propulsion, primarily by segmentation
- Chemical digestion of carbohydrates, fats, polypeptides, nucleic acids
- Absorption of peptides, amino acids, glucose, fructose, fats, water, minerals, and vitamins

- Mechanical digestion includes segmental mixing and propulsion
- No chemical digestion (except by bacteria)
- Absorption of ions, water, minerals, vitamins, and organic molecules

Esophagus

Liver

Gallbladder

Pylorus

Pancreas

Rectum

Anal sphincter

Openstax College courses.candelalearning.com Creative Commons License

Much like the water hoses and spray that greet your vehicle as you enter the beginning of the car wash tunnel, the entrance of food to the mouth receives a similar welcome. Jets of saliva are secreted from the ducts of the salivary glands located strategically around the oral cavity of the mouth. Saliva that is in the resting mouth is viscous and coats and protects the teeth and the inner surface of the mouth. The secreted saliva with eating or drinking is of a thinner more watery consistency. It has digestive enzymes including amylase to digest carbohydrates and lipase to digest fats.

If your carwash is as sophisticated as your digestive tract, it will have a crew to make sure your side mirrors are tucked in, and a prewash scrub of your tires and residue that would otherwise be difficult for the machinery to come. The teeth, jaws, and tongue work together in a remarkable and powerful dance with very few of the missteps which would be the dance equivalent of stepping on toes, the biting of the tongue.

The food has to be processed into smaller more manageable portions than that what is found on your plate. Your dining utensils of fork, knife, and spoon are just the preliminary, as the teeth do the real work in preparing food for the process of digestion. The teeth are subdivided into specific categories that have unique functions.

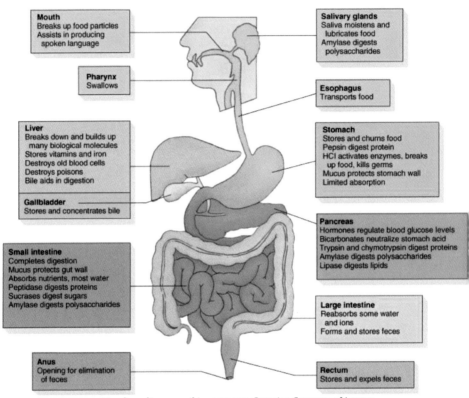

peptic-ulcer-disease-wikispaces.com Creative Commons License

The incisors cut the food as you bite into an apple, the canines tear the food apart as you dig into your pastrami sandwich, and your molars crush and grind the salad and crunchy vegetables you have as a side dish. The grinding and crushing break the plant cell walls apart that would otherwise protect its internal nutritious content from our digestive enzymes. They also increase the surface area of the food increasing their exposure to digestive acid and enzymes.

The chewing process assures that the saliva and its active enzymes are well mixed with the increased surface area of the food. They begin the process of breaking down the carbohydrates and lipids into their essential components to ready them for further digestion and absorption. The saliva also moistens the food and lubricates it for the coordinated swallowing motion of the tongue, teeth, palate and pharynx. These muscles and organs work together to roll it into an easy to swallow food bolus. The muscles of the swallowing process include those that protect the larynx and airway. By having the epiglottis close off the passageway to the trachea, bronchi, and lungs, it prevents aspiration into the airways as the food and saliva swallow takes place.

The coordinated action is developed with age, which is why small children should avoid foods, such as nuts, grapes, larger oval or rounded candies. These foods, if inappropriately swallowed into the airway, can lead to fatal choking episodes. Tragically a number of children die because the oval or rounded shape can completely block the airway. An irregular shaped object, which can be life threatening, rarely completely obstructs the airway and usually allows some air to pass.

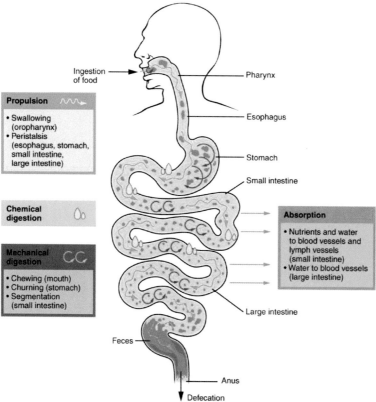

Openstax College philschatz.com Creative Commons License

The complicated swallowing neuromuscular coordination can also be affected by neurological disorders, stroke, surgery or other conditions, which may lead to the risk of aspiration. Once swallowed, the food bolus is propelled down the esophagus by coordinated snakelike muscular action, known as peristalsis. It is not recommended, but the swallowing mechanism is so effective that you can swallow against gravity while standing on your head.

The muscular valve at the junction of the esophagus and stomach is called the lower esophageal sphincter. The lower esophageal sphincter is designed to allow food and fluid to enter the stomach, with the door closed behind them once they leave the esophagus. If the valve opens at the wrong time, gastric acid, digestive enzymes, and food can flow back into the esophagus. This can lead to symptoms of heartburn or mucosal damage. If the refluxed material goes all the way into the airway hoarseness, sore throat, aspiration, choking, or pneumonia can develop. If it occurs frequently gastroesophageal reflux disease (GERD) can predispose to a change in the tissue lining the esophagus. The growth of intestinal type tissue is called a Barrett esophagus, and is at a higher risk of cancer development than the normal lining tissue. Individuals with Barrett esophagus are treated for GERD and monitored closely for pre-malignant changes.

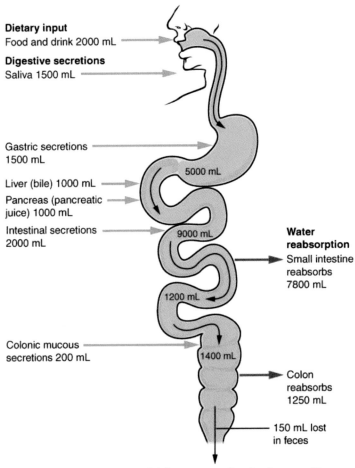

Dietary input
Food and drink 2000 mL

Digestive secretions
Saliva 1500 mL

Gastric secretions
1500 mL

5000 mL

Liver (bile) 1000 mL
Pancreas (pancreatic juice) 1000 mL

Intestinal secretions
2000 mL

9000 mL

Water reabsorption
Small intestine reabsorbs
7800 mL

1200 mL

Colonic mucous
secretions 200 mL

1400 mL

Colon reabsorbs
1250 mL

150 mL lost in feces

Openstax College courses.candelalearning.com Creative Commons License

The stomach is a churning cauldron of muscular mixing contractions, concentrated acid secretion, and potent digestive enzymes. The Vagus nerve and gut hormones play a key role in the intricate balance of enzymes, acid, nutrients, and motility. When the conditions are right, the pyloric sphincter of the stomach opens to allow the acid, enzyme, and food mixture to exit. This digestive material is now called chyme as it enters the first portion of the small intestine, known as the duodenum. In Greek, this means the width equivalent to twelve fingers, which is what its small size would measure using your digits. For its small size, the duodenum plays an amazing and complex part.

The highly acidic chyme would quickly damage the lining of the duodenum if it did not respond quickly with the pouring on, much like a fire extinguisher, of sodium bicarbonate. The sodium bicarbonate is produced in the duodenum itself, as well as the pancreas. The sodium bicarbonate produced in the pancreas is released through the pancreatic duct, which empties into the duodenum through the Ampulla of Vater.

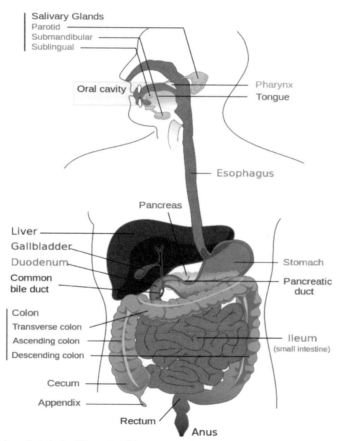

Mariana Ruiz LadyofHats, edited by Joaquim Alves Gaspar Creative Commons License

The fire extinguisher analogy shares another aspect of the story. Perhaps you made a fire extinguisher in a science class, or home experiment, by adding baking soda that contains sodium bicarbonate and vinegar that contains acetic acid. This is the same type of reaction that takes place in the duodenum, when the hydrochloric acid of the stomach meets the sodium bicarbonate released to neutralize it. When the two react they produce water, sodium chloride (salt), and large quantities of carbon dioxide. The carbon dioxide is released as large volumes of gas that appears as a bubbles arising from the reaction. The carbon dioxide is used as a fire extinguisher in the science experiment since it is heavier than air, and cuts off the oxygen supply that the fire requires. In the human duodenum, the carbon dioxide generated as a side product of acid neutralization only serves to bloat and distend the gut with gas. The body is pretty remarkable in getting rid of the bloat fairly quickly, in that it absorbs the carbon dioxide into the bloodstream where it travels to the lungs to be exhaled.

Major Digestive Enzymes

Enzyme	Produced In	Site of Release	pH Level
Carbohydrate Digestion:			
Salivary amylase	Salivary Glands	Mouth	Neutral
Pancreatic amylase	Pancreas	Small Intestine	Basic
Maltase	Small intestine	Small intestine	Basic
Protien Digestion:			
Pepsin	Gastric glands	Stomach	Acidic
Trypsin	Pancreas	Small intestine	Basic
Peptidases	Small Intestine	Small intestine	Basic
Nucleic Acid Digestion:			
Nuclease	Pancreas	Small intestine	Basic
Nucleosidases	Pancreas	Small intestine	Basic
Fat Digestion:			
Lipase	Pancreas	Small intestine	Basic

commons.wikimedia.org Creative Commons License

The bile ducts from the liver join the duct from the pancreas bringing digestive enzymes and bicarbonate that enter the duodenum through the Ampulla of Vater. Within the ampulla lies the muscular sphincter of Oddi. The name sounds like a character from the story of the Wizard of Oz, and that would be an appropriate analogy. The coordinated release of hormones, enzymes, motility and vagal input is nothing short of wizardry. Subconsciously, your body can sense exactly what nutrients you have ingested. It responds by releasing the best recipe of enzymes, acid in the stomach, and bicarbonate in the duodenum, adjusting the pH as necessary. It adds just the right amount of bile to the mix, controls the timing and volume of stomach emptying, and controls the speed of transit and intensity of mixing contractions through the length of the intestinal tract. The majority of the sensing and control feedback takes place in a small confined space the width of twelve fingers, the duodenum.

The breakdown products of the digestive process are absorbed through a sea of finger like projections called the villi. It looks like a field of waving wheat stalks, each upstanding villus is ready to use its enzymes and absorptive capacity to absorb nutrients. If you looked under the microscope you would find that each villus has thousands of even smaller villi on its surface, given the appropriate name of microvilli. All of these folds of absorptive tissue, if flattened out, would provide the equivalent absorptive capacity of a championship tennis court. A quote from Mark Twain also illustrates the concept of surface area: "If Switzerland were ironed flat it would be a very large country". The long intestinal tunnel of eagerly awaiting absorptive villi is about twenty feet long, and it is an amazingly efficient system of digestion and absorption.

If injured, the ability of the small bowel to digest and absorb nutrients is compromised. A condition that temporarily damages the small intestine, such as a viral or bacterial gastroenteritis often called stomach flu, can cause a blunting or shortening of the villi. The villous blunting will also lead to the loss of digestive enzymes that reside on the villi. Without the ability to digest and absorb nutrients, the unabsorbed material can cause what is known as an osmotic diarrhea. This is one of the reasons people are often advised to avoid dairy products for a week or so after stomach flu to allow the villi and enzymes to recover. If you eat or drink lactose without waiting until the recovery is complete, you may end up with symptoms of temporary lactose intolerance such as gas and diarrhea.

When the liquid chyme leaves the jejunum and ileum of the small intestine, it goes through the ileocecal valve to enter the colon. In the cecum of the colon lies the infamous appendix, which for thousands of years mystified science as to its purpose. It looks like its function has finally, and only very recently, been identified. It stores a reservoir of intestinal bacteria, representing the healthy gut microbiome, from which the gut flora can be replenished after a bout of intestinal dysentery.

The gut microbiome is much more important than most people give it credit for. The microbes of the body far outnumber the number of human cells. In fact, if you simply go by the number of cells and not their mass, they outnumber human cells by ten to one. In other words, you as a living system are only ten percent human, and ninety percent microbes! The vast majority of the microbes living within and on us are commensals. This means that they are engaged with us in a symbiotic relationship from which we both benefit. They are able to process foods that would otherwise be indigestible, and convert them to absorbable nutrients and metabolites. It is not an understatement to say that they are a requirement for our health and wellbeing. The gut microbiome also plays a very important role in the gut-brain-microbiome-axis, which provides for the communication of important information between the three. Many experts now include food as the fourth component of this important communication axis.

The colon, unlike the small intestine, is less involved in the digestion of foods and nutrients. It is primarily involved in the absorption of water and sodium, as well as some fat-soluble vitamins such as vitamin K. The colon removes the excess moisture from the watery chyme, and the stool solidifies as it transits the gut. The ability to conserve water is very important, and without this ability the risk of dehydration would be substantially increased. The fecal material of the stool is stored in the rectum and sigmoid colon awaiting the right opportunity to be eliminated through defecation.

A process or illness that impairs the colon's absorption of water will lead to more fluid in the stool and diarrhea. The loss of water and electrolytes as a consequence of diarrhea unfortunately remains a life threatening condition in many parts of the world, especially for infants and children. If the elimination of the feces is delayed, the moisture continues to be absorbed and the stools can become harder resulting in constipation. Constipation itself can be self-perpetuating as it aggravates the situation because the stools become harder and more difficult to pass the longer they remain in the colon. The more common treatments for constipation attempt to increase the moisture content of the stool.

The feces excreted can provide information about bowel health. For most people going about their daily activities, the passage of the feces itself is the end of the story of digestion. The human digestive system, like that of other animals, does not remove all of the available nutrients from food. For other organisms, including the common housefly, the feces are thus an available source of nutrition. For them the elimination of feces is just the beginning of their story of digestion, and can play an important role in the transmission of disease back to humans.

Continued from Volume One

VIII. Chronology of Fart in Literature

Bel-Phegor

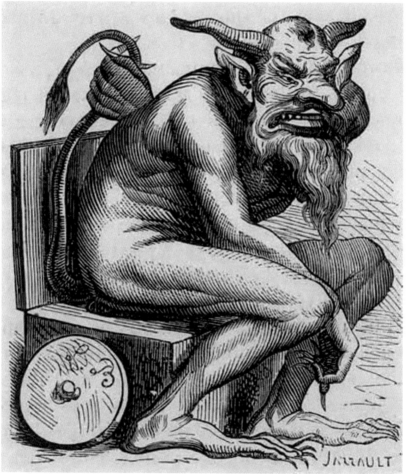

Illustration of Bel-Phegor in De Plancy's *Dictionnaire Infernal* Public Domain

The ancient Pelusians of northern Egypt worshipped the god called Bel-Phegor with farts and bowel movements as religious offerings. More details of their practices are included in the work *Scatological Rites of All Nations* referenced under the entry for John Bourke. "The ancient Pelusiens, a people of lower Egypt, did (amongst other whimsical, chimerical objects of veneration and worship) venerate a Fart, which they worshipped under the symbol of a swelled paunch." — ("*A View of the Levant*," Charles Perry, M. D., sm. fob, London, 1743, p. 419.

Bel-Phegor is considered one of the seven princes of hell in demonology. He is thought to have been derived from the Assyrian Baal-Peor and was considered a god by the Moabites. He is referenced in John Milton's *Paradise Lost* and in Victor Hugo's *The Toilers of the Seas.*

Aristophanes

Aristophanes (c. 446 BCE – c. 386 BCE) was a comical playwright of Ancient Greece. His 5th century BC plays The Knights and The Clouds, which contain numerous fart jokes.

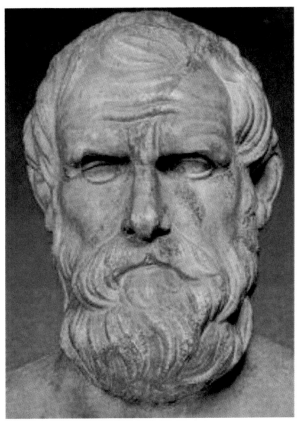

Aristophanes Public Domain

The Clouds: " First, think of a tiny fart that your intestines make. Then consider the heavens: their infinite farting is thunder. For thunder and farting are, in principle, one and the same.

Strepsiades: By Apollo, of a truth you have rightly confirmed this by your present argument. And yet, before this, I really thought that Jupiter caused the rain. But tell me who is it that thunders. This makes me tremble.

Socrates: These, as they roll, thunder.

Strepsiades: In what way? you all-daring man!

Socrates: When they are full of much water, and are compelled to be borne along, being necessarily precipitated when full of rain, then they fall heavily upon each other and burst and clap.

Strepsiades: Who is it that compels them to borne along? Is it   not Jupiter?

Socrates: By no means, but aethereal Vortex.

Strepsiades: Vortex? It had escaped my notice that Jupiter did not exist, and that Vortex now reigned in his stead. But you have taught me nothing as yet concerning the clap and the thunder.

Socrates: Have you not heard me, that I said that the Clouds, when full of moisture, dash against each other and clap by reason of their density?

Strepsiades: Come, how am I to believe this?

Socrates: I'll teach you from your own case. Were you ever, after being stuffed with broth at the Panathenaic festival, then disturbed in your belly, and did a tumult suddenly rumble through it?

Strepsiades: Yes, by Apollo! And immediately the little broth plays the mischief with me, and is disturbed and rumbles like thunder, and grumbles dreadfully: at first gently pappax, pappax; and then it adds papa-pappax; and finally, it thunders downright papapappax, as they do.

Socrates: Consider, therefore, how you have trumpeted from a little belly so small; and how is it not probable that this air, being boundless, should thunder so loudly?

Strepsiades: For this reason, therefore, the two names also Trump and Thunder, are similar to each other. But teach me this, whence comes the thunderbolt blazing with fire, and burns us to ashes when it smites us, and singes those who survive. For indeed Jupiter evidently hurls this at the perjured.

Socrates: Why, how then, you foolish person, and savouring of the dark ages and antediluvian, if his manner is to smite the perjured, does he not blast Simon, and Cleonymus, and Theorus? And yet they are very perjured. But he smites his own temple, and Sunium the promontory of Athens, and the tall oaks. Wherefore, for indeed an oak does not commit perjury.

Strepsiades: I do not know; but you seem to speak well. For what, pray, is the thunderbolt?

Socrates: When a dry wind, having been raised aloft, is inclosed in these Clouds, it inflates them within, like a bladder; and then, of necessity, having burst them, it rushes out with vehemence by reason of its density, setting fire to itself through its rushing and impetuosity.

Strepsiades: By Jupiter, of a truth I once experienced this exactly at the Diasian festival! I was roasting a haggis for my kinsfolk, and through neglect I did not cut it open; but it became inflated and then suddenly bursting, befouled my eyes and burned my face.

Plutus:

My wind exploded like a thunderclap,
Iaso flushed a rosy red,
And Panacea turned away her head,
Holding her nose:
My wind's no frankincense.

The Frogs: First performed at Lenea in 405 BCE
Translated by George Theodoridis © 2008, used with permission

Xanthias: (Frowns. Shifts his load again and again the donkey farts) Well... what about – can't I even say the one about how... what about the one about how... "I'm carrying such a burden on my shoulders that if someone doesn't give me some relief I'll start farting?

Dionysus:
No! I beg you! Please! Not that one either! At least not until I'm ready to puke.

Xanthias:
Then what's the point of carrying this huge burden if I can't do what all the others do? Your competitors, boss: Phrynicus and Lycis and Ameipsias! That's how they always win the comedy prize, by carrying burdens and...

Petronius

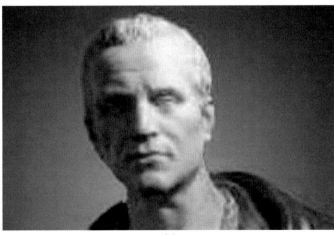

Gaius Petronius Arbiter (c. 27 – 66 AD) was a Roman courtier during the reign of Nero. He is the author of *Satyricon*, a satirical novel.

"Take my word for it, friends, the vapors go straight to your brain. Poison your whole system. I know some who have died from being too polite and holding it in".

Famous Quotations:

"We trained hard—but it seemed that every time we were beginning to form up into teams we were reorganized. I was to learn later in life that we tend to meet any new situation by reorganizing, and what a wonderful method it can be for creating the illusion of progress while actually producing confusion, inefficiency, and demoralization."

Marcus Valerius Martialis

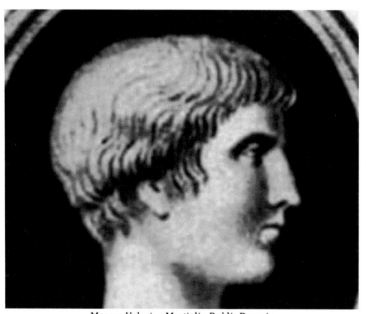

Marcus Valerius Martialis, Public Domain

Marcus Valerius Martialis was known in English as Martial (40 AD – c. 104 AD). He was a Latin poet from the region of Hispania on the Iberian Peninsula. He is considered to be the creator of the modern short and witty epigram. He also humorously satirized city life and the scandalous activities of its citizenry.

While Aethon was praying in the Capitol, with many a supplication, to Jupiter, and with up-turned eyes was bowing to his very feet, he let wind escape behind. The bystanders laughed, but the father of the gods was offended, and condemned his worshipper to dine at home for three successive days.

After this accident, the unhappy Aethon, when he wished to enter the Capitol, goes first to Patroclus' house of convenience, and relieves himself by some ten or twenty discharges. But, notwithstanding this precaution, he is careful never to address Jove again without being tightly compressed in the rear.

Fabullus' wife Bassa frequently totes
A friend's baby, on which she loudly dotes.
Why does she take on this childcare duty?
It explains farts that are somewhat fruity.

Matthew's mouth smells like an arse,
To scientist's great confusion.
Without a label none can parse
The source of his effusions.
When he speaks of love, or art -
All his listeners think he farts.

Famous Quotations:

"Be content with what you are, and wish not change; nor dread your last day, nor long for it."
"Joys do not stay, but take wing and fly away."
 "Fortune gives too much to many, enough to none."
"Conceal a flaw, and the world will imagine the worst ."
"A man who lives everywhere, lives nowhere."
"If fame is to come after death, I am in no hurry for it."
"Tomorrow's life is too late. Live today."
"Virtue extends our days. He live two lives who relives his past with pleasure."
"Life is not merely being alive, but being well."

Arabian Nights

The stories and essays collected over hundreds of years under various titles was first called *The Book of the Tales of the Thousand Nights* with the earliest manuscript dating to the 9th century. The first European translation was into French in 1704 and comprised twelve volumes.

Captain Sir Richard Francis Burton (1821 – 1890) was an English geographer, translator, orientalist, explorer, translator, cartographer, writer, and diplomat. soldier, ethnologist, spy, linguist, poet, and fencer. He was known for his extraordinary facility and knowledge of languages and cultures. He insinuated himself into the heart of Arabic culture and was one of the few westerners who travelled to Mecca incognito. He was the translator of *The Arabian Nights*, and related the tale of the unforgettable fart of Abu al-Hassan, The Merchant of Oman tale.

"He let fly two great farts, one of which blew up the dust from the earth's face and the other steamed up the gates of Heaven." Abu – al-Hassan upon his wedding night "let fly a fart, great and terrible". He was so ashamed he ran from house and went into exile for ten years. When re returned, hoping that his fart was long forgotten he overheard a mother telling her child she "was born on the very night that Abu al-Hassan farted!" Mortified that his fart had become a landmark day in the history of his people he returned to exile never to return gain.

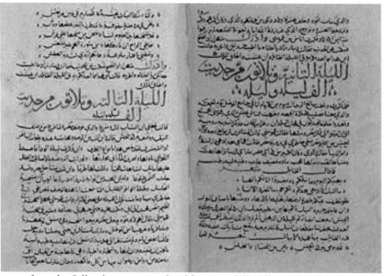

Two pages from the Galland manuscript, the oldest text of *The Thousand and One Nights*. Arabic manuscript, back to the 14th century. Public Domain

Another version of these folk tales was compiled and published as *The Book of the Thousand Nights and One Night* in 1923 by Edward Powys Mathers. The story that follows was entitled *The Father of Farts*.

That morning the girl prepared a dish consisting of beans, peas, white haricots, cabbage, lentils, onions, and cloves of garlic, various heavy grains and powdered spices. The qadi's enormous belly was quite empty when he returned for the midday meal, so he took helping after helping of this mixture, until all was finished...

The qadi congratulated himself, as he had so often done before, on the excellent choice of a wife; but an hour afterwards his belly began visibly to swell. A noise as of a far-off tempest made itself heard inside him. Low grumblings and far thunders shook the walls of his being and brought in their train sharp colics, spasms, and a final agony. He grew yellow in the face and began to roll groaning about the floor, holding his belly in his two hands.

"Allah, Allah!" he cried. "I have a terrible storm within! Who will deliver me?" Soon his paunch became as tight as a gourd, and his cries brought his wife running. She made him swallow a powder of anise and fennel, which was soon to have its effect, and, at the same time, to console and encourage him, began rubbing and patting the afflicted part, as if he had been a little sick child…

Then his pains increased, and he fell howling to the floor in a crisis of agony. Suddenly came relief. A long and thunderous fart broke from him, shaking the foundations of the house and throwing its utterer violently forward, so that he swooned. Then followed a multitude of other escapes, gradually diminishing in sound but rolling and re-echoing through the troubled air. Last came a single deafening explosion, and all was still.

Dante Alighieri

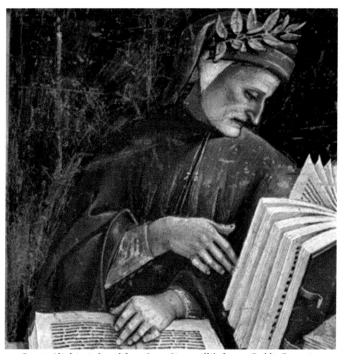

Dante Alighieri, detail from Luca Signorelli's fresco, Public Domain

Durante degli Alighieri (c. 1265 – 1321) wrote in his famous work, *Divine Comedy*, the last line of Inferno Chapter XXI: ed elli avea del cul fatto trombetta. In other words: "and he used his buttocks as a trumpet."

And more graphically yet in Canto XXVIII, Circle Eight, Bolgia Nine, the Sowers of Discord, "A wine tun when a stave or cant-bar starts does not split open as wide as one saw split from his chin to the mouth with which man farts. Between his legs all of his red guts hung with the heart, the lungs, the liver, the gall bladder, and the shriveled sac that passes shit to the bung.

Famous Quotations:

"The wisest are the most annoyed at the loss of time."
"The hottest places in hell are reserved for those who, in times of great moral crisis, maintain their neutrality."
He who sees a need and waits to be asked for help is as unkind as if he had refused it."
"A mighty flame follows a tiny spark."
"Nature is the art of God."

The Divine Comedy:
"All hope abandon, ye who enter here."

Inferno:
"Ye who enter, abandon all hope."

Paradise:
"My course is set for an uncharted sea."

Rutebeuf

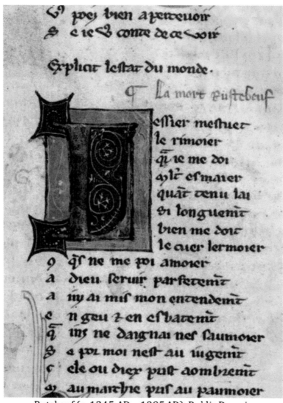

Rutebeuf (c. 1245 AD – 1285 AD), Public Domain

Rutebeuf (c. 1245 AD – 1285 AD) was an author and satirist using a pen name (nome de plume) and is roughly translated as 'coarse ox'. In *The Peasant's Fart* he addresses the effects of food in relation to social class.

The peasant's digestive upsets are caused by his diet, but the devil persuades him to believe that his fart is his soul leaving his body. The devil convinces the peasant to trap his fart in a bag and release it in Hell.

William Langland

William Langland (1332-1386) is the most likely author of the classic English poem *Piers Plowman*. Along with Chaucer's *Canterbury Tales* t is considered one of the finest works of English literature in the Middle Ages. It is an allegorical tale as well as social satire.

The character Activa Vita has the ability to fart as a means of entertainment and is critical to the success of traveling performers. "As for me, I can neither drum nor trumpet, nor tell jokes, nor fart amusingly at parties, nor play the harp."

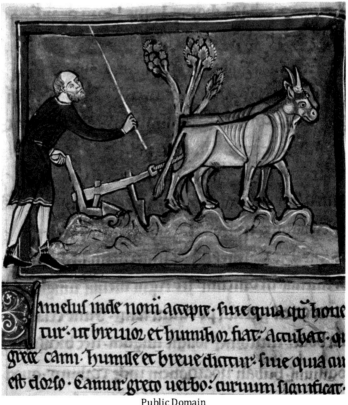

Public Domain

Famous Quotations:

"Necessity has no law "
"There smites nothing so sharp, nor smelleth so sour as shame"
"But all the wickedness in the world which man may do or think is no more
to the mercy of God than a live coal dropped in the sea."
"When all treasures are tried...truth is the fairest."

Geoffrey Chaucer

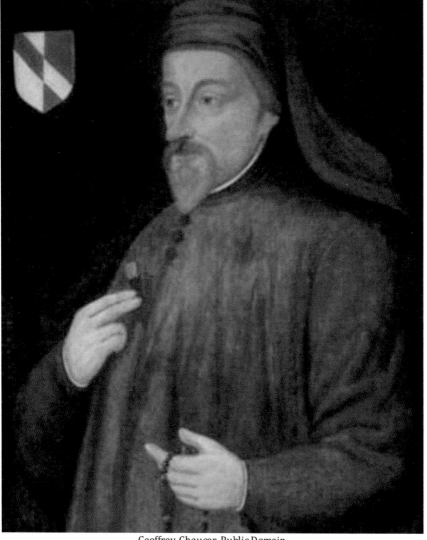

Geoffrey Chaucer, Public Domain

Geoffrey Chaucer (c. 1343-1400) was a master storyteller, one of his most famous tales is that of *The Millers Wife*. One of the humorous scenes is where a lover climbs a ladder in the dark of night to visit an attractive lady he is trying to woo. Another fellow has already beaten him to her bedroom and when the latecomer climbs the ladder and asks for a cheek that he may kiss, the other fellow presents him the cheek of his butt.

In the dark the latecomer bestows a kiss and is so happy that he asks for her to blow a kiss back. What he blows back came from between his cheeks as a fart.

"Sing, sweet bird, I kneen nat where thou art!
This Nicholas anon leet fle a fart
As greet as it had been a thonder-dent,
That with the strook he was almoost y blent;
And he was redy with his iren hoot,
And Nicholas amydde the ers he smoot.
Of gooth the skyn an hande-brede aboute,
The hoote kultour brende so his toute,
And for the smert he wende for to dye."

The original Middle English may be difficult to understand at first. Following the portrait of the author below is a brief section of the prologue in the original Middle English followed by a modern English translation.

THE MILLER'S PROLOGUE (in Middle English)
Whan that the knyght had thus his tale ytoold,
In al the route nas ther yong ne oold
That he ne seyde it was a noble storie,
And worthy for to drawen to memorie;
And namely the gentils everichon.
Oure hooste lough and swoor, so moot I gon,
This gooth aright; unbokeled is the male.
Lat se now who shal telle another tale;
For trewely the game is wel bigonne.
Now telleth ye, sir monk, if that ye konne
Somwhat to quite with the knyghtes tale.
The millere, that for dronken was al pale,
So that unnethe upon his hors he sat,
He nolde avalen neither hood ne hat,
Ne abyde no man for his curteisie,
But in pilates voys he gan to crie,
And swoor, by armes, and by blood and bones,
I kan a noble tale for the nones,
With which I wol now quite the knyghtes tale.

THE MILLER'S PROLOGUE (in Modern English)
The Words between the Host and the Miller
Now when the knight had thus his story told,
In all the rout there was nor young nor old
But said it was a noble story, well
Worthy to be kept in mind to tell;
And specially the gentle folk, each one.
Our host, he laughed and swore, "So may I run,
But this goes well; unbuckled is the mail;
Let's see now who can tell another tale:
For certainly the game is well begun.
Now shall you tell, sir monk, if't can be done,
Something with which to pay for the knight's tale."
The miller, who with drinking was all pale,
So that unsteadily on his horse he sat,
He would not take off either hood or hat,
Nor wait for any man, in courtesy,
But all in Pilate's voice began to cry,
And by the Arms and Blood and Bones he swore,
"I have a noble story in my store,
With which I will requite the good knight's tale."

Famous Quotations:

"The life so brief, the art so long in the learning, the attempt so hard, the conquest so sharp, the fearful joy that ever slips away so quickly - by all this I mean love, which so sorely astounds my feeling with its wondrous operation, that when I think upon it I scarce know whether I wake or sleep."
"What is better than wisdom? Woman. And what is better than a good woman? Nothing."
"All that glitters is not gold,"
"The greatest scholars are not usually the wisest people"
"Nothing Ventured, Nothing Gained"
"How potent is the fancy! People are so impressionable, they can die of imagination."
"Life is short. Art long. Opportunity is fleeting. Experience treacherous. Judgment difficult."
"Forbid Us Something and That Thing we Desire"
"Patience is a conquering virtue."
"Time and Tide wait for no man"

François Rabelais

François Rabelais (1494 – 1553) is the author of the *Tales of Gargantua and Pantagruel*. Both of these tales are filled with farts and ribald humor.

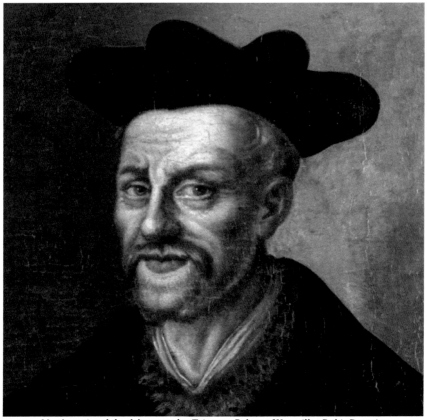

Musée national du château et des Trianons Palace of Versailles Pubic Domain

In Chapter XXVII of the second book, the giant, Pantagruel "made the earth shake for twenty-nine miles around, and the foul air he blew out created more than fifty-three thousand tiny men, dwarves and creatures of weird shapes, and then he emitted a fat wet fart that turned into just as many tiny stooping women."

Gargantua and Pantagruel:

"He would sit down between two stools: cover himself with a wet sock, spin in the basin and fart for fatness." (Referring to Gargantua)

Famous Quotations:

"We always long for the forbidden things, and desire what is denied us"
"Science without conscience is the soul's perdition."
"I have nothing, I owe a great deal, and the rest I leave to the poor."
"I am going to seek a great perhaps; bring down the curtain, the farce is played

out." (His last words before dying)

"Readers, friends, if you turn these pages
Put your prejudice aside,
For, really, there's nothing here that's outrageous,
Nothing sick, or bad — or contagious.
Not that I sit here glowing with pride
For my book: all you'll find is laughter:
That's all the glory my heart is after,
Seeing how sorrow eats you, defeats you.
I'd rather write about laughing than crying,
For laughter makes men human, and courageous."

John Heywood

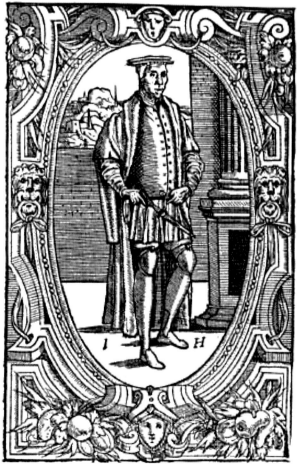

John Heywood. Public Domain

John Heywood (c. 1497 – c. 1580) was an English author, poet, composer, musician, and playwright.

"They're as nervous as a fart in a mitten lookin for a thumb hole"?

What wind can there blow that doth not some man please? A fart in the blowing doth the blower ease.

Famous Quotations:

"A man may well bring a horse to the water but he cannot make him drink."
"Rome was not built in one day."
"Two heads are better than one."
"Nothing is impossible to a willing heart"
"Would ye both eat your cake and have your cake?"
"Enough is as good as a feast."
"Every dog has its day!!"

William Shakespeare

William Shakespeare (1564 - 1616) was an English poet and playwright, and is regarded by many experts as the greatest writer in the English language. Shakespeare was careful not to use the word fart or flatus itself but there is no question that he is referring to farting in several scenes.

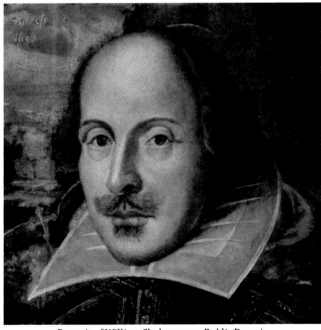

Portrait of William Shakespeare, Public Domain

In *Henry IV*, Part I, Act III:

Hotspur: O, then the earth shook
to see the heavens on fire,
And not in fear of your nativity.
Diseased nature oftentimes breaks forth
In strange eruptions; oft the teeming earth
Is with a kind of colic pinch'd and vex'd
By the imprisoning of unruly wind
Within her womb; which,
for enlargement striving,
Shakes the old beldam earth and topples down
Steeples and moss-grown towers.
At your birth Our grandam earth,
having this distemperature,
In passion shook.

Macbeth, Act I, Scene III

Second Witch: I'll give thee a wind.

First Witch: Thou'rt kind.

Third Witch: And I another.

First Witch: I myself have all the other,
And the very ports they blow,
All the quarters that they know
I' the shipman's card.
I will drain him dry as hay:
Sleep shall neither night nor day
Hang upon his pent-house lid;
He shall live a man forbid:
Weary se'nnights nine times nine
Shall he dwindle, peak and pine:
Though his bark cannot be lost,
Yet it shall be tempest-tost.
Look what I have.

In *Othello*, Act IV, Scene I:

Clown: Why masters, have your instruments been in
Naples, that they speak i' the nose thus?

First Musician: How, sir, how!

Clown: Are these, I pray you, wind-instruments?

First Musician: Ay, marry, are they, sir.

Clown: O, thereby hangs a tail.

First Musician: Whereby hangs a tale, sir?

Clown: Marry. sir, by many a wind-instrument that I
            know.   But, masters, here's money for you:
            and the general so likes your music,
            that he desires you,

In *Comedy of Errors*, Act III

'A man may break a word with you, sir; and words are but wind; Ay, and break it in your face, so he break it not behind.'

Shakespeare also uses a pun to refer to the podex, the arse musica, as a 'wind-instrument'

Famous Quotations:

"You speak an infinite deal of nothing."
"With mirth and laughter let old wrinkles come."
"Conscience doth make cowards of us all."
"Some are born great, others achieve greatness."
"All's well if all ends well."
"Thou of thyself thy sweet self dost deceive."
"Better a witty fool, than a foolish wit."
"The best is yet to come."
"Foul words is but foul wind, and foul wind is but foul breath, and foul breath is noisome; therefore I will depart unkissed."
"Who knows himself a braggart, let him fear this, for it will come to pass that every braggart shall be found an ass."
"Ambition should be made from sterner stuff."
"I love you with so much of my heart that none is left to protest."
"The sweetest honey is loathsome in its own deliciousness. And in the taste destroys the appetite. Therefore, love moderately."
"When I got enough confidence, the stage was gone. When I was sure of losing, I won. When I needed people the most, they left me. When I learnt to dry my tears, I found a shoulder to cry on. And when I mastered the art of hating, somebody started loving me."
"My dull brain was wrought with things forgotten."
"By my soul I swear, there is no power in the tongue of man to alter me."
"That which we call a rose, by any other name would smell as sweet"

"Set your teeth on edge"
"Too much of a good thing"
"Wear your heart on your sleeve"
"What's done is done"
"Love is blind"
"Vanish into thin air"
"They are the books, the arts, the academes,
That show, contain and nourish all the world."
"Off with his head"
"The world is my oyster"
"Come what may"
"The game is up"
"Makes your hair stand on end"
"Break the ice"
"Not slept one wink"
"Brave new world"
"A piece of work"
"Green eyed monster"
"Out of the jaws of death"
"Dead as a doornail"
"Be all, end all"
"Baited breath"
"Full circle"
"Fight fire with fire"
"Faint hearted"
"Send him packing"
"Seen better days"
"Men from children nothing differ."
"Laughing stock"
"Wild goose chase"
"Lie low"
"Fair play, foul play"
"Heart of hearts"
"Breathed his last"
"A sorry sight"
"In a pickle"
"Naked truth"
"Heart of gold"
"For goodness sake"
"Good riddance"
"So-so"
"Be as thou wast wont to be.
See as thou wast wont to see."

"To be, or not to be: that is the question:
Whether 'tis nobler in the mind to suffer

The slings and arrows of outrageous fortune,
Or to take arms against a sea of troubles,
And by opposing end them? To die: to sleep;
No more; and by a sleep to say we end
The heart-ache and the thousand natural shocks
That flesh is heir to, 'tis a consummation
Devoutly to be wish'd. To die, to sleep;
To sleep: perchance to dream: ay, there's the rub;
For in that sleep of death what dreams may come
When we have shuffled off this mortal coil,
Must give us pause: there's the respect
That makes calamity of so long life;"

Francois Béroalde de Verville

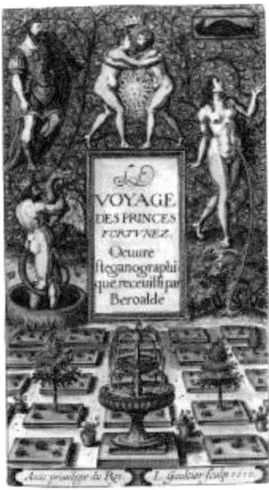

Le Voyage des princes fortunez, Beroalde de Verville. Public Domain

Francois Béroalde de Verville (1556 – 1626) was a French Renaissance poet, novelist, and intellectual. Writing in *Moyen de Parvenir* in 1610 tells a ribald tale dealing with aromatic farts.

I'll clinch the matter by telling you the story of what happened to a French gentleman, the Sieur of Lierne, when he lay with a gay lady of Rome.

She, after the fashion of her chaste sisterhood, had a store of little light pellicles or bladders, soft dainty things and filled with sweet musk-scented perfume. And with sundry of these little balloons secreted about her, the fair Imperia – that was her name – lay with the gentleman in her arms and let him love her.

While the two of them were toying with the dainties of love and savouring its keen delights, the lady with a cunning twist of her hand slipped one of her little bladders high up near the place of state, and then with a tiny press of her thigh burst it. The gentleman, hearing the report, wished to take his nose out of bed to get some fresh air. "'Tis not what you think," said Imperia; "one should know the worst before one begins to be afraid."

At this persuasion the gentleman put his head back and met with a delicious odour and one quite different from what he had expected. This pleasant trick having occurred several times, he asked the lady if such sweet smelling airs came natural to her, seeing that those which floated around the lower parts of French ladies were of quite another kind.

She replied with a philosophic frisk that the natural air of the country and the aromatic delicacies upon which the Italian ladies fed were distilled inside 'em and issued quintessential from the breech, as from the beak of an alchemist's retort. "Very surely," said he, "our French ladies' wind blows from a different quarter." – However, it happened that after several more these musk(et) shots, Imperia, by force of a superfluity of internal wind, let a real fart, a highly natural, solid and substantial one.

The Frenchman, whose nose had got into the habit of chasing after these reports (from whence cometh the saying: to lead by the nose), hearing the short, sharp crack, quickly burrowed his diligent proboscis under the sheets, so as to catch every fragment of the sweet breeze for the better apprehension of which he had wished himself made all nose.

But alas! he was mistaken, and he drew back his nose quicker than you could have done it for him with forty of those great wooden shovels they measure corn with at Orleans. Wherefore? He had met with a smell so shocking, coming from the very heart of the bad place, that none before or since had smelt its peer.

"Oh lady," quoth he sadly, "what have you done?" And as he opened his mouth to say this, in leapt that warm breeze and played across his palate. "Sir," laughed she, "'tis a compliment to remind you of your native land and loved ones far away!"

Famous Quotation:

"Laughter for the soul, and wine for the body."

Ben Jonson

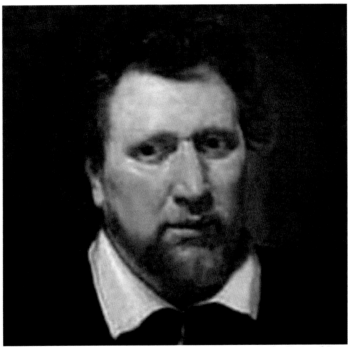

Ben Jonson (c.1617), by Abraham Blyenberch; oil on canvas painting at the National Portrait Gallery, London. Public Domain

Benjamin Jonson (1572 – 1637) was an English playwright and poet whose work had a significant impact on English literature. He was a contemporary of William Shakespeare, and enjoyed a reputation for being controversial.

In *The Alchemist*:
I fart at thee.
And then my poets,
The same that writ so subtly of the fart.
In *The Pranks of Robin Goodfellow*:

Then, lads and lasses, merry be,
With possets and with juncates fine,
Unseen of all the company,

I eat their cakes and sip their wine;
And, to make sport,
I fart and snort.
And out the candles I do blow.

Volpone in *The Fox*:
These turdy-facy-nasty-paty-lousy-fartical
rogues, with one poor groat's-worth of unprepared
antimony, finely wrapt up in several scartoccios,^ are
able, very well, to kill their twenty a week, and play.

On the Famous Voyage (his mock-epic of a journey down the Fleet Ditch, then an
open sewer)
Here, sev'ral Ghosts did flit
About the shore, of Farts, but late departed,
White, Black, Blue, Green, and in more Forms out-started,
Than all those Atomi Ridiculous,
Whereof old Democrite, and Hill Nicholas,
One said, the other swore, the World consists.
These be the cause of those thick frequent Mists
Arising in that place, through which, who goes,
Must try th' unused Valor of a Nose.

Famous Quotations:

"To speak and to speak well, are two things. A fool may talk, but a wise man
speaks."
"True happiness consists not in the multitude of friends, but in the worth and
choice."
"He knows not his own strength that has not met adversity."
"Good men are the stars, the planets of the ages wherein they live, and illustrate
the times."
"Success produces confidence; confidence relaxes industry, and negligence ruins
the reputation which accuracy had raised."
"There is no greater hell than to be a prisoner of fear."
"Language most shows a man, speak that I may see thee."
"He that is taught only by himself has a fool for a master."
"Let them call it mischief: When it is past and prospered t'will be virtue."
"Honor's a good brooch to wear in a man's hat at all times."
"Talking and eloquence are not the same: to speak, and to speak well, are two
things."
"They that know no evil will suspect none."
"Weigh the meaning and look not at the words."
"O, for an engine, to keep back all clocks, or make the sun forget his motion!"

43

"In small proportions we just beauties see; And in short measures, life may perfect be."

"Tis no shame to follow the better precedent."

"No man is so foolish but he may sometimes give another good counsel, and no man so wise that he may not easily err if he takes no other counsel than his own. He that is taught only by himself has a fool for a master."

"Cares that have entered once in the breast, will have whole possession of the rest."

"Art has an enemy called ignorance."

"Talking is the disease of age."

"That for which all virtue is now sold,
And almost every vice – almighty gold."

John Donne

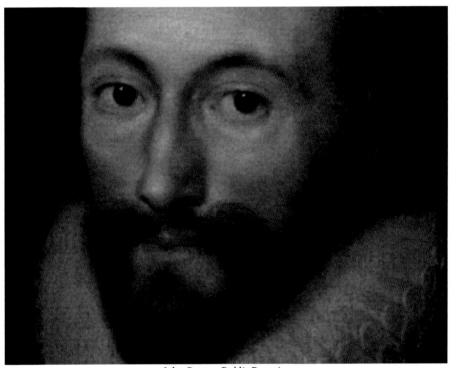

John Donne, Public Domain

John Donne (1572-1631) was an English poet and cleric. He is considered one of the pre-eminent metaphysical poets of the English language.

The Courtier's Library:
The notrhingness of the fart

Satyre 2:

hee is worst, who (beggarly) doth chaw,
Others wits fruits, and in his ravenous maw
Rankly digested, those things out-spue,
As his owne things; and they are his owne, 'tis true,
For if one eate my meate, though it be known
The meate was mine, th'excrement is his owne..

Famous Quotations:

"Be thine own palace, or the world's thy jail."
"No spring nor summer beauty hath such grace as I have seen in one autumnal
face."
"I am two fools, I know,
For loving, and for saying so."
"And who understands? Not me, because if I did I would forgive it all."
"More than kisses, letters mingle souls."
"To know and feel all this and not have the words to express it makes a human a
grave of his own thoughts."
"Love, built on beauty, soon as beauty, dies."
"Hee that hath all can have no more"
"Death be not proud, though some have called thee mighty and dreadful, for, thou
art not so."

"No man is an island, entire of itself; every man is a piece of the continent, a part
of the main. If a clod be washed away by the sea, Europe is the less, as well as if a
promontory were, as well as if a manor of thy friend's or of thine own were: any
man's death diminishes me, because I am involved in mankind, and therefore
never send to know for whom the bells tolls; it tolls for thee."

"Come live with me, and be my love,
And we will some new pleasures prove
Of golden sands, and crystal brooks,
With silken lines, and silver hooks."

Sir John Suckling

Sir John Suckling (1609-1642) was an esteemed poet of the early 17th Century. He
also invented the popular card game of cribbage

'Love is the fart
Of every heart;
It pains a man when
'tis kept close
And others doth offend
when 'tis let loose.'

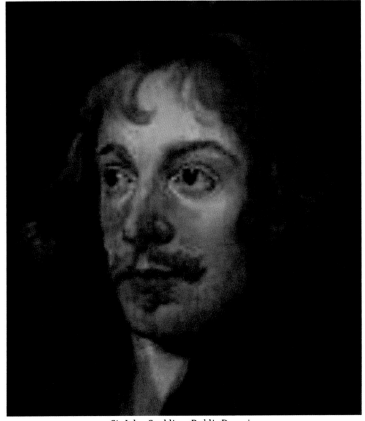

Sir John Suckling, Public Domain

Anther Famous Poem:
"I prithee send me back my heart,
Since I cannot have thine;
For if from yours you will not part,
Why, then, shouldst thou have mine?"

John Milton

John Milton (1608-1674) was an English poet and author whose most famous work was *Paradise Lost*, authored when he was blind and impoverished. He sold the rights for a nominal sum but regained his wealth with further writings. He was influential in the political and religious debates of his era.

In *Paradise Lost* he makes reference to Bel-Phegor. The ancient Pelusians of northern Egyptian's worshipped the god called Bel-Phegor with farts and bowel movements as religious offerings. More details of their practices is included in the work *Scatological Rites of All Nations* (see entry on John Bourke).

" The ancient Pelusiens, a people of lower Egypt, did (amongst other whimsical, chimerical objects of veneration and worship) venerate a Fart, which they worshipped under the symbol of a swelled paunch." — (*A View of the Levant* by Charles Perry, M. D., London, 1743, p. 419. Bel-Phegor is considered one of the seven princes of hell in demonology. He is thought to have been derived from the Assyrian Baal-Peor and was considered a god by the Moabites.

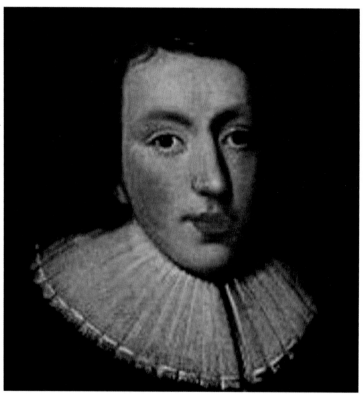

Portrait of John Milton, Public Domain

Famous Quotations:

"Innocence, Once Lost, Can Never Be Regained. Darkness, Once Gazed Upon, Can Never Be Lost."
"Such sweet compulsion doth in music lie."

Paradise Lost:
"The mind is its own place, and in itself can make a heaven of hell, a hell of heaven.."
"Solitude sometimes is best society."

Areopagitica:
"For books are not absolutely dead things, but do contain a potency of life in them

to be as active as that soul was whose progeny they are; nay, they do preserve as in a vial the purest efficacy and extraction of that living intellect that bred them."

Comus
"Thou canst not touch the freedom of my mind."

John Aubrey

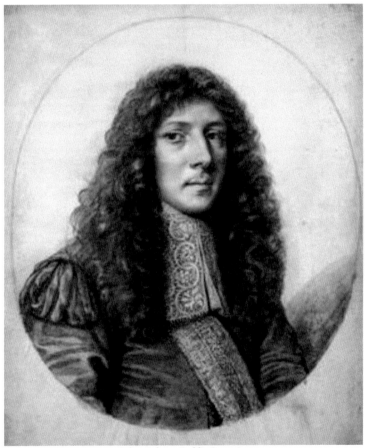

John Aubrey, Public Domain

John Aubrey (1626-1697) was a biographer and antiquary who described the story of the seventeenth Earl of Oxford, Edward de Vere (1550-1604) in his volume *Brief Lives*.

"This Earl of Oxford, making of his low obeisance to Queen Elizabeth, happened to let a Fart, at which he was so abashed and ashamed that he went to travel for seven years. On his return the Queen welcomed him home, and said, "My Lord, I had forgotten the Fart".

Daniel Defoe

Daniel Defoe (1660 – 1731) was an English author, journalist and spy. Defoe is one of the earliest practitioners of the English novel. A prolific and versatile writer, he wrote on various topics including politics, crime, religion, marriage, psychology and the supernatural. His most famous for his novel *Robinson Crusoe*. In *The History of The Devil* he describes the devil as calling "Religion itself flatus".

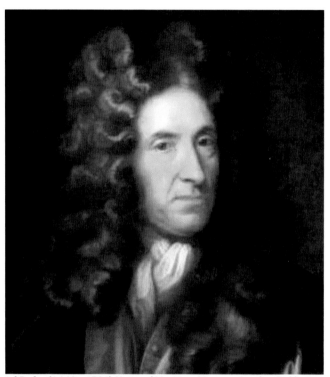

Daniel Defoe (1660 – 1731) National Maritime Museum, London Public Domain

He himself had a very colorful history of scandal including a major bankruptcy due to investing in civet cats to harvest their anal glands to create a perfume. Although that may sound like a bizarre enterprise, many are surprised to find that the scent glands of the musk dear are prized for their use in perfumes.

The musk scent glands are not true anal glands, but are in the general area of the animal's reproductive and excretory organs. Another interesting feature of the civet cat is their propensity to harvest and digest coffee beans at their peak ripeness.

The coffee beans are harvested from the civet cat droppings, thankfully washed, roasted and then marketed as the exclusive Kopi Luwak (civet coffee). This product originated in Indonesia and is the most expensive coffee in the world, with a characteristic mellow flavor attributed to the digestive enzymes of the civet digestive tract.

Famous Quotations:

"It is never too late to be wise."

"Expect nothing and you'll always be surprised"

"Thus fear of danger is ten thousand times more terrifying than danger itself when apparent to the eyes ; and we find the burden of anxiety greater, by much, than the evil which we are anxious about : ..."

"He that hath truth on his side is a fool as well as a coward if he is afraid to own it because of other men's opinions."

"Those people cannot enjoy comfortably what God has given them because they see and covet what He has not given them. All of our discontents for what we want appear to me to spring from want of thankfulness for what we have."

"I hear much of people's calling out to punish the guilty, but very few are concerned to clear the innocent."

Lord John Wilmot Earl of Rochester

Lord John Wilmot (1647 - 1680) Earl of Rochester was an English poet and satirist whose writings were frequently censored during the Victorian period.

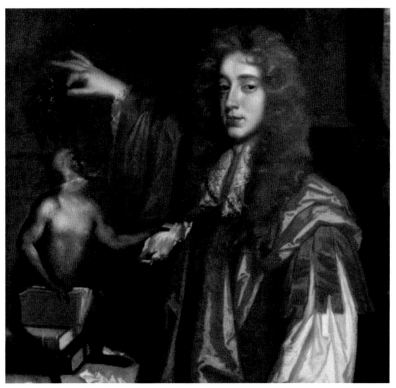

Lord John Wilmot, Earl of Rochester Public Domain

He is the author of the following epistle:
Perhaps ill Verses, ought to be confined,
In mere good Breeding, like unsavory wind.
Were Reading forced, I should be apt to think
Men might no more write scurvily than stink.
But 'tis your choice, whether you'll read or no;
If likewise of your smelling it were so,
I'd Fart, just as I write, for my own ease,
Nor should you be concerned unless you please.

Jonathan Swift

Jonathan Swift (1667 – 1745) was an Anglo Irish author, essayist, satirist, and cleric. The pamphlet *The Benefit of Farting Explained* was published under the pseudonym Don Fartinando Puff-Indorst, Professor of Bumbast at the University of Crackow. The actual author was Jonathan Swift, the famed author of *Gulliver's Travels*, with numerous references to farting, borborygmi, and gastrointestinal bodily functions.

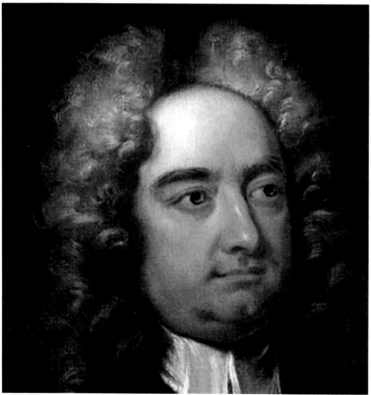

Jonathan Swift, Public Domain

He was considered the most brilliant satirist in the English language in the 18th Century. Other contemporaries considered him certifiably insane for partaking in such scatological endeavors. This is particularly unusual in that he was a well established cleric and was dean of St. Patrick's Cathedral of the Church of Ireland.

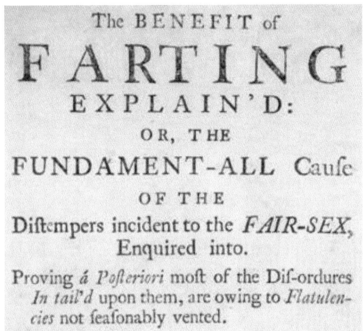

The BENEFIT of

FARTING

EXPLAIN'D:

OR, THE

FUNDAMENT-ALL Caufe

OF THE

Diftempers incident to the *FAIR-SEX*, Enquired into.

Proving *á Pofteriori* moft of the Dif-ordures *In tail'd* upon them, are owing to *Flatulen-cies* not feafonably vented.

The Benefit of Farting Explain'd Or, The Fundament-All Cause of the Distempers incident to the Fair-Sex, enquired into. Proving á Posteriori most of the Dis-ordures In tail'd upon them, are owing to Flatulen-cies not seasonably vented. Wrote in Spanish by Don Fartinando Puff-indorst', Professor of Bumbast in the University of Crackow. And Translated into English at the Request, and for the Use, of the Lady Damp - fart of Her-fart-shire. By Obadiah Fizzle, Groom of the Stool to the Princess of Arsimini in Sardinia. Long-Fart (Longford in Ireland): Authored by Jonathon Swift under an assumed pen name. Public Domain

Swift describes four types of farts, and how to produce them. They are:
First, *the sonorous and full-toned, or rousing fart;*
Second, *the double fart;*
Third, *the soft fizzing fart;*
And fourth, *the sullen wind-bound fart.*

"Fart away, then, my brethren, and let farting be in common among you. Vie with each other in producing ... the sonorous, full-toned, loud fart."

He also composed poems of an equal scatological bent

"A Fart, tho' wholesome, does not fail
   If barr'd of Passage by the Tail,

To fly back to the Head again,
And, by its Fumes, disturb the Brain:
Thus Gunpowder confin'd, you know, Sir,
Grows stronger, as 'tis ram'd the closer;
But if in open Air it fires,
In harmless Smoke its Force expires."

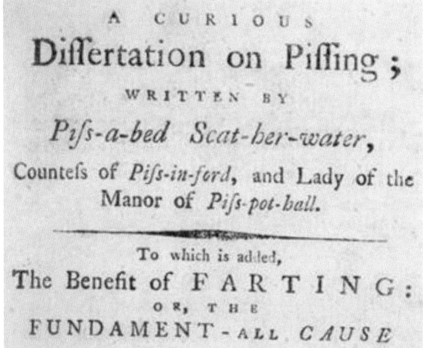

Benefits, A Curious Dissertation on Pissing; Written by Piss-A-Bed Scat-Her-Water, Countess of Piss-in-Ford, and Lady of the Manor of Piss-Pot-Hall. 1787 Authored by Jonathon Swift under an assumed pen name. Public Domain

"THAT MY LORD BERKELEY STINKS WHEN HE IS IN LOVE"
Did ever problem thus perplex,
Or more employ the female sex?
So sweet a passion who would think,
Jove ever form'd to make a stink?
The ladies vow and swear, they'll try,
Whether it be a truth or lie.
Love's fire, it seems, like inward heat,
Works in my lord by stool and sweat,
Which brings a stink from every pore,
And from behind and from before;
Yet what is wonderful to tell it,
None but the favourite nymph can smell it.
But now, to solve the natural cause

By sober philosophic laws;
Whether all passions, when in ferment,
Work out as anger does in vermin;
So, when a weasel you torment,
You find his passion by his scent.
We read of kings, who, in a fright,
Though on a throne, would fall to sh--.
Beside all this, deep scholars know,
That the main string of Cupid's bow,
Once on a time was an a-- gut;
Now to a nobler office put,
By favour or desert preferr'd
From giving passage to a t--;
But still, though fix'd among the stars,
Does sympathize with human a--.
Thus, when you feel a hard-bound breech,
Conclude love's bow-string at full stretch,
Till the kind looseness comes, and then,
Conclude the bow relax'd again.
And now, the ladies all are bent,
To try the great experiment,
Ambitious of a regent's heart,
Spread all their charms to catch a f--
Watching the first unsavoury wind,
Some ply before, and some behind.
My lord, on fire amid the dames,
F--ts like a laurel in the flames.
The fair approach the speaking part,
To try the back-way to his heart.
For, as when we a gun discharge,
Although the bore be none so large,
Before the flame from muzzle burst,
Just at the breech it flashes first;
So from my lord his passion broke,
He f--d first and then he spoke.
The ladies vanish in the smother,
To confer notes with one another;
And now they all agreed to name
Whom each one thought the happy dame.
Quoth Neal, whate'er the rest may think,
I'm sure 'twas I that smelt the stink.
You smell the stink! by G--d, you lie,
Quoth Ross, for I'll be sworn 'twas I.
Ladies, quoth Levens, pray forbear;
Let's not fall out; we all had share;
And, by the most I can discover,

My lord's a universal lover.

Voltaire

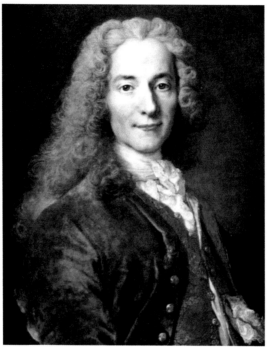

Voltaire, Public Domain

François-Marie Arouet (1694 – 1778) was known by his pen name (*nom de plume*) of Voltaire. He lived during the period of the French Enlightenment and was a celebrated writer, philosopher, and historian. He had a very sharp wit and used satirical writings to challenge religious dogma and called for the separation of church and state.

"Inspiration: A peculiar effect of divine flatulence emitted by the Holy Spirit which hisses into the ears of a few chosen of God..."

Crepitus was described as the Roman god of flatulence but probably was a fiction created to denigrate Roman theology. He appears as a god in several works of French literature by Voltaire, Charles Baudelaire, and Gustave Flaubert as well as material promoting Roman Catholicism as the true faith.

Famous Quotations:

"Let us read, and let us dance; these two amusements will never do any harm to the world."
"Life is a shipwreck, but we must not forget to sing in the lifeboats."

"The more I read, the more I acquire, the more certain I am that I know nothing."

"Judge a man by his questions rather than by his answers."

"Those who can make you believe absurdities, can make you commit atrocities."

"Love truth, but pardon error."

"Now, now my good man, this is no time to be making enemies."
(Voltaire on his deathbed in response to a priest asking him that he renounce Satan.)"

"The secret of being a bore is to tell everything."

"The most important decision you make is to be in a good mood."

"It is dangerous to be right in matters on which the established authorities are wrong."

"Every man is guilty of all the good he did not do."

"God is a comedian playing to an audience that is too afraid to laugh."

"Dare to think for yourself."

"Faith consists in believing what reason cannot."

"I do not agree with what you have to say, but I'll defend to the death your right to say it."

"Think for yourself and let others enjoy the privilege of doing so too."

"If God did not exist, it would be necessary to invent him."

"Doubt is an uncomfortable condition, but certainty is a ridiculous one."

"I don't know where I am going, but I am on my way."

"Fools have a habit of believing that everything written by a famous author is admirable. For my part I read only to please myself and like only what suits my taste."

"The human brain is a complex organ with the wonderful power of enabling man to find reasons for continuing to believe whatever it is that he wants to believe."

"Prejudices are what fools use for reason."

"Every man is a creature of the age in which he lives and few are able to raise themselves above the ideas of the time."

"We never live; we are always in the expectation of living."

"The comfort of the rich depends upon an abundant supply of the poor."

"What is history? The lie that everyone agrees on..."

"The art of medicine consists of amusing the patient while nature cures the disease."

"Men will always be mad, and those who think they can cure them are the maddest of all."

"No opinion is worth burning your neighbor for."

"Don't think money does everything or you are going to end up doing everything for money."

"It is with books as with men: a very small number play a great part."

"Animals have these advantages over man: they never hear the clock strike, they die without any idea of death, they have no theologians to instruct them, their last moments are not disturbed by unwelcome and unpleasant ceremonies, their funerals cost them nothing, and no one starts lawsuits over their wills."

"The only way to comprehend what mathematicians mean by Infinity is to contemplate the extent of human stupidity."

"Liberty of thought is the life of the soul."

"It is clear that the individual who persecutes a man, his brother, because he is not of the same opinion, is a monster."

"Men are equal; it is not birth but virtue that makes the difference."

"May God defend me from my friends: I can defend myself from my enemies. "

"The longer we dwell on our misfortunes, the greater is their power to harm us"

"Behind every successful man stands a surprised mother-in-law."

"One great use of words is to hide our thoughts."

"To succeed in the world it is not enough to be stupid - one must also be polite."

"Good is the enemy of great."

"History never repeats itself. Man always does."

"Opinions have caused more ills than the plague or earthquakes on this little globe of ours. "

"With great power comes great responsibility"

"If you have two religions in your land, the two will cut each other's throats; but if you have thirty religions, they will dwell in peace"

"Meditation is the dissolution of thoughts in Eternal awareness or Pure consciousness without objectification, knowing without thinking, merging finitude in infinity."

"When it is a question of money, everybody is of the same religion."

"The discovery of what is true and the practice of that which is good are the two most important aims of philosophy."

"Each player must accept the cards life deals him or her; but once they are in hand, he or she alone must decide how to play the cards in order to win the game."

"It is not inequality which is the real misfortune, it is dependence."

"What can you say to a man who tells you he prefers obeying God rather than men, and that as a result he's certain he'll go to heaven if he cuts your throat?"

"There is a wide difference between speaking to deceive, and being silent to be impenetrable."

"In general, the art of government consists in taking as much money as possible from one party of the citizens to give to the other."

"Doctors put drugs of which they know little into bodies of which they know less for diseases of which they know nothing at all."

"It is hard to free fools from the chains they revere."

"Being unable to make people more reasonable, I preferred to be happy away from them"

"The greatest consolation in life is to say what one thinks."

"If there's life on other planets, then the earth is the Universe's insane asylum."

"Is politics nothing other than the art of deliberately lying?"

"Life is thickly sown with thorns, and I know no other remedy than to pass quickly through them. The longer we dwell on our misfortunes, the greater is their power to harm us."

"No problem can stand the assault of sustained thinking."

"I have chosen to be happy because it is good for my health."

"Uncertainty is an uncomfortable position. But certainty is an absurd one."

"The more a man knows, the less he talks."

"God gave us the gift of life; it is up to us to give ourselves the gift of living well."

"To believe in God is impossible not to believe in Him is absurd."

"A witty saying proves nothing."

"The man who leaves money to charity in his will is only giving away what no longer belongs to him"

"Wherever my travels may lead, paradise is where I am."

"Religion began when the first scoundrel met the first fool."

"To find out who rules over you, simply find out who you are not allowed to criticize."

"I have seen so many extraordinary things that nothing seems extraordinary to me"

"God's only excuse is that He doesn't exist," remarked Voltaire after a natural disaster that killed many people. Nietzsche loved this quote and wished he'd coined it!"

"All our ancient history, as one of our wits remarked, is no more than accepted fiction."

"Christianity is the most ridiculous, the most absurd, and bloody religion that has ever infected the world."

"Originality is nothing but judicious imitation"

"A witty saying proves nothing"

"Common sense is not so common"

"The only thing necessary for the triumph of evil is for good people to do nothing."

Henry Fielding

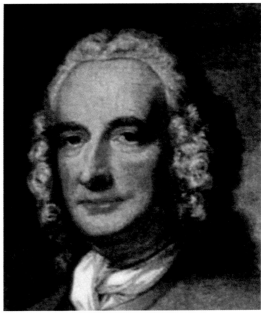

Henry Fielding, Public Domain

Henry Fielding (1707-1754) was an English novelist and magistrate known for his earthy sense of humor and satire as seen in his novel *The History of Tom Jones*. Also attributed to him is a controversial play that was published to promote limiting censorship in the theater, *The Golden Rump*. In the *History of Tom Jones, a Foundling* Fielding used "f—t" in place of the word fart to circumvent censors.

Famous Quotations:

"I am content; that is a blessing greater than riches; and he to whom that is given need ask no more."
"We are as liable to be corrupted by books as we are by companions."
"One fool at least in every married couple."

The History of Tom Jones, a Foundling:

"And here, I believe, the wit is generally misunderstood. In reality, it lies in desiring another to kiss your a-- for having just before threatened to kick his; for I have observed very accurately, that no one ever desires you to kick that which belongs to himself, nor offers to kiss this part in another."
"It is much easier to make good men wise, than to make bad men good."
"Men are strangely inclined to worship what they do not understand. A grand secret, upon which several imposers on mankind have totally relied for the success of their frauds."

Jean Anthelme Brillat-Savarin

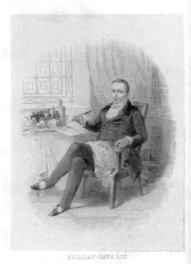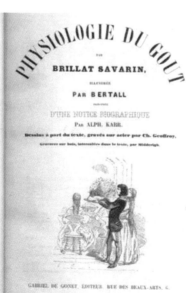

Brillat Savarin, Public Domain

Jean Anthelme Brillat-Savarin (1755-1826) was a French gastronome, politician, lawyer, and author of *Physiologie du goût* (The Physiology of Taste, 1825).

From *Physiologie du goût* (The Physiology of Taste, 1825): "The intestines are the home of tempests; in them is formed gas, as in the clouds; oxygen is found in them, whilst the fat producers hydrogen and carbon.

The foods of the animal kingdom give nitrogen; an unknown process generates sulfur and phosphorus, and hence those emissions of sulphureted hydrogen of which the effects are known by every one, but which the author is never known."

Famous Quotations:

"Tell me what you eat, and I will tell you what you are."
"The discovery of a new dish does more for the happiness of the human race than the discovery of a star."
"The fate of a nation depends on the way that they eat."
"Those who have been too long at their labor, who have drunk too long at the cup of voluptuousness, who feel they have become temporarily inhumane, who are tormented by their families, who find life sad and
love ephemeral......they should all eat chocolate and they will be comforted."
"Burgundy makes you think of silly things, Bordeaux makes you talk of them and Champagne makes you do them."
"Food is all those substances which, submitted to the action of the stomach, can be assimilated or changed into life by digestion, and can thus repair the losses which the human body suffers through the act of living."

William Blake

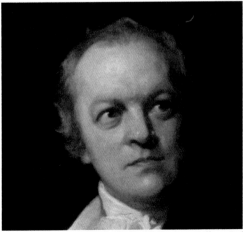

William Blake Artist Thomas Phillips National Portrait Gallery Public Domain

William Blake (1757 – 1827) was an English poet and artist.

In *When Klopstock England Defied* :
When Klopstock England defied,
Uprose William Blake in his pride;
For old Nobodaddy aloft
. . . and belch'd and cough'd;
Then swore a great oath that made Heaven quake,
And call'd aloud to English Blake.
Blake was giving his body ease,
At Lambeth beneath the poplar trees.
From his seat then started he
And turn'd him round three times three.
The moon at that sight blush'd scarlet red,
The stars threw down their cups and fled,
And all the devils that were in hell,
Answerнd with a ninefold yell.
Klopstock felt the intripled turn,
And all his bowels began to churn,
And his bowels turn'd round three times three,
And lock'd in his soul with a ninefold key; . . .
Then again old Nobodaddy swore
He ne'er had seen such a thing before,
Since Noah was shut in the ark,
Since Eve first chose her hellfire spark,
Since 'twas the fashion to go naked,
Since the old Anything was created . . .

Famous Quotations:

"What is now proved was once only imagined."
 "The imagination is not a state: it is the human existence itself."
"A man can't soar too high, when he flies with his own wings."
"The hours of folly are measur'd by the clock, but of wisdom: no clock can measure."
"The man who never alters his opinion is like standing water, and breeds reptiles of the mind."
"In seed time learn, in harvest teach, in winter enjoy."
"We become what we behold."
 "none can desire what he has not perceiv'd."
"Knowledge is Life with wings"
"Enlightenment means taking full responsibility for your life."

Johann Wolfgang Von Goethe

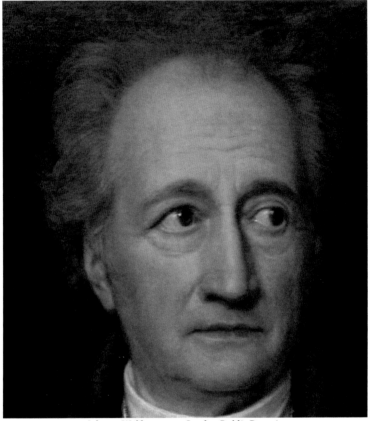

Johann Wolfgang von Goethe Public Domain

Johann Wolfgang von Goethe (1749 – 1832) was a brilliant German author, artist, philosopher, and politician. His prolific and critically acclaimed writings made him one of the most influential individuals of all time. Many of his writings were set to music.

In *Faust Part I*
Translation by A.S. Kline @ 2003

Witches: (In chorus.)
To Brocken's tip the witches stream,
The stubble's yellow, the seed is green.
There the crowd of us will meet.
Lord Urian has the highest seat.
So they go, over stone and sticks,
The stinking goat, the farting witch.

Famous Quotations:

"To tremble before anticipated evils is to bemoan what thou hast never lost."
"If one has not read the newspapers for some months and then reads them all together, one sees, as one never saw before, how much time is wasted with this kind of literature."
"Mistrust all those in whom the desire to punish is imperative."
"Science and art belong to the whole world, and before them vanish the barriers of nationality."
"I am fully convinced that the soul is indestructible, and that its activity will continue through eternity. It is like the sun, which, to our eyes, seems to set in night; but it has in reality only gone to diffuse its light elsewhere."
"If you treat an individual as he is, he will remain how he is. But if you treat him as if he were what he ought to be and could be, he will become what he ought to be and could be."
"In the realm of ideas, everything depends on enthusiasm.... In the real world, all rests on perseverance."
"There is no crime of which I do not deem myself capable."
"Whatever you can do or dream you can, begin it. Boldness has genius, power and magic in it!"
"We do not have to visit a madhouse to find disordered minds; our planet is the mental institution of the universe."
"You can easily judge the character of a man by how he treats those who can do nothing for him."
"By seeking and blundering we learn."
"Nothing shows a man's character more than what he laughs at."
"I love those who yearn for the impossible."
"We must always change, renew, rejuvenate ourselves; otherwise, we harden."
"knowing is not enough, we must apply
   willing is not enough, we must do.."
"Everything is hard before it is easy"
"The intelligent man finds everything laughable, the sensible man hardly anything."
"Rest not, Life is sweeping by
go and dare before you die.
Something mighty and sublime,
leave behind to conquer time."
"Whatever you can do, or dream you can, begin it."
"In all things it is better to hope than to despair."
"It's irrelevant whether what one says is true or false: both will be contradicted."
"Nothing is worse than active ignorance."
"None are so hopelessly enslaved as those who falsely believe they are free."
"A rainbow which lasts for a quarter of an hour is looked at no longer."
"The moment one definitely commits oneself, then Providence moves too. All sorts of things occur to help one that would never otherwise have occurred. A whole stream of events issues from the decision which no man could have

63

dreamed would have come his way. Whatever you can do, or dream you can do, begin it. Boldness has genius, power, and magic in it. Begin it now."
"If we put ourselves in the place of other people, the jealousy and hatred we so often feel about them would disappear, and if we put others in our place, pride and conceit would greatly diminish."
"Doubt grows with knowledge."
"Just begin and the mind grows heated; continue, and the task will be completed!"
"There are two things children should get from their parents: roots and wings."
 "What is not started today is never finished tomorrow."

"It is ever true that he who does nothing for others, does nothing for himself."
"Treat people as if they were what they ought to be and you help them to become what they are capable of being."
"He who moves not forward, goes backward."
"He is happiest, be he king or peasant, who finds peace in his home."
"The highest goal that man can achieve is amazement."
"Misunderstandings and neglect occasion more mischief in the world than malice and wickedness."
"Oblivion is full of people who allow the opinions of others to overrule their belief in themselves."
"Who is the happiest of men? He who values the merits of others, and in their pleasure takes joy, even as though 'twere his own. "
"Too many parents make life hard for their children by trying, too zealously, to make it easy for them."
"Doubt can only be removed by action."
"We know accurately only when we know little; doubt grows with knowledge."
 "What you get by achieving your goals is not as important as what you become by achieving your goals."
"Music is liquid architecture; Architecture is frozen music."
"One never goes so far as when one doesn't know where one is going."
"Divide and rule, a sound motto. Unite and lead, a better one."
 "If you don't feel it, you'll never get it."
"At the moment of commitment the entire universe conspires to assist you."
"Know thyself? If I knew myself, I'd run away."
"A person hears only what they understand."
None are more hopelessly enslaved than those who falsely believe they are free."
"It is not doing the thing we like, but liking the thing we have to do that makes life happy."
"There is nothing more frightful than ignorance in action."

Jacques Collin de Plancy

Jacques Collin de Plancy (1793-1881) was a French author and occultist who was a free thinker influenced by Voltaire. He authored and published *Dictionnaire Infernal* describing the ancient god Bel-Phegor, worshipped with farts and bowel movements, as Hell's ambassador to France.

The ancient god Bel-Phegor is referenced in Victor Hugo's The Toilers of the Seas. The ancient Pelusians of northern Egyptian's worshipped the god called Bel-Phegor with farts and bowel movements as religious offerings. Bel-Phegor is considered one of the seven princes of hell in demonology. He is thought to have been derived from the Assyrian Baal-Peor and was considered a god by the Moabites.

More details of their practices are included in the work *Scatological Rites of All Nations* referenced under John Bourke later in this chapter. "The ancient Pelusiens, a people of lower Egypt, did (amongst other whimsical, chimerical objects of veneration and worship) venerate a Fart, which they worshipped under the symbol of a swelled paunch." — ("A View of the Levant," Charles Perry, M. D., sm. fob, London, 1743, p. 419.

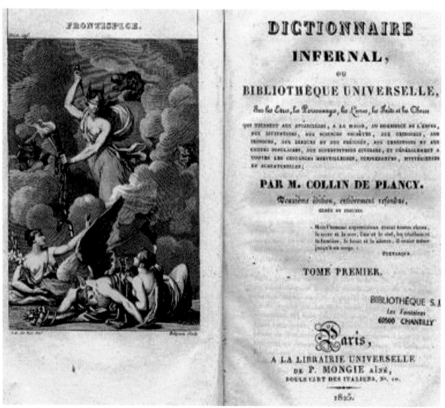

Dictionnaire Infernal by Jacques Collin de Plancy Public Domain

Honoré de Balzac

Honoré de Balzac (1799–1850) was a French novelist and playwright was a keen observer of French life, particularly in the years after the fall of Napoleon

Bonaparte in 1815. Balzac openly described his desire for fame and notoriety in an unusual manner. He stated that he wanted to be "so well known, so popular, so celebrated, so famous, that it would.... permit me to break wind in society and society would think it a most natural thing."

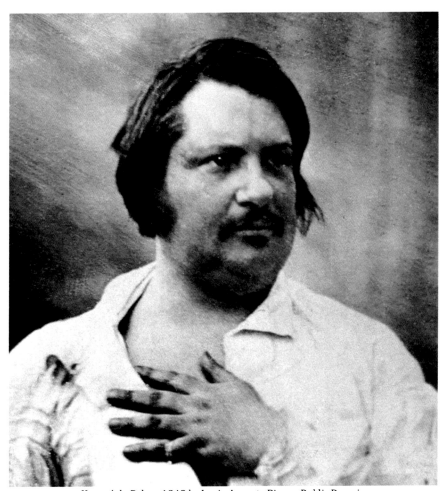

Honoré de Balzac 1842 by Louis-Auguste Bisson. Public Domain

With his detailed and unfiltered view of society he is regarded as one of the pioneers of realism in French literature. Some considered his work vulgar with a focus on bodily functions and filth, especially in his series called *The Droll Stories*.

Famous Quotations:

"Our worst misfortunes never happen, and most miseries lie in anticipation."
"Bureaucracy is a giant mechanism operated by pygmies."
"Behind every great fortune there is a crime."

Victor Hugo

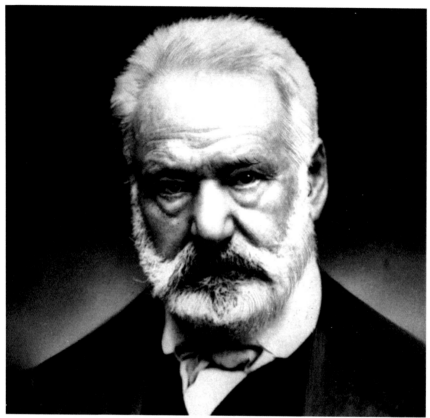

Victor Hugo, Public Domain

Victor Marie Hugo (1802 – 1885) was a French poet, novelist, and dramatist. A scene in Victor Hugo's *The Hunchback of Notre Dame* is based on an actual custom that was a well known requirement of the working women in question during the fourteenth and fifteenth Centuries.

Prostitutes of the day were required to "make a payment of a fart when they crossed the toll bridge at Montluc".

"Abbé Claude Choart! Doctor Claude Choart! Are you in search of Marie la Giffarde?"
"She is in the Rue de Glatigny."
"She is making the bed of the king of the debauchees." She is paying her four deniers.
"*Or one explosion (fart)*"
"Would you like to have her pay you through the nose?"

The ancient god Bel-Phegor is referenced in Victor Hugo's *The Toilers of the Seas*. The ancient Pelusians of northern Egyptian's worshipped the god called Bel-Phegor with farts and bowel movements as religious offerings. Bel-Phegor is considered one of the seven princes of hell in demonology. He is thought to have been derived from the Assyrian Baal-Peor and was considered a god by the Moabites.

More details of their practices are included in the work *Scatological Rites of All Nations* referenced under John Bourke later in this chapter. " The ancient Pelusiens, a people of lower Egypt, did (amongst other whimsical, chimerical objects of veneration and worship) venerate a Fart, which they worshipped under the symbol of a swelled paunch." — (*A View of the Levant* by Charles Perry, M.D., sm. fob, London, 1743, p. 419.

Bel-Phegor was considered Hell's ambassador to France in De Plancy's *Dictionairre Infernal*.

Famous Quotations:

"A garden to walk in and immensity to dream in--what more could he ask? A few flowers at his feet and above him the stars."
"As with stomachs, we should pity minds that do not eat."
"Now life has killed the dream I dreamed."
"Never, even among animals, does the creature born to be a dove change into an osprey. That is only seen among men."

"So long as there shall exist, by virtue of law and custom, decrees of damnation pronounced by society, artificially creating hells amid the civilization of earth, and adding the element of human fate to divine destiny; so long as the three great problems of the century—the degradation of man through pauperism, the corruption of woman through hunger, the crippling of children through lack of light—are unsolved; so long as social asphyxia is possible in any part of the world;—in other words, and with a still wider significance, so long as ignorance and poverty exist on earth, books of the nature of Les Misérables cannot fail to be of use.

"Let no one misunderstand our idea; we do not confound what are called 'political opinions' with that grand aspiration after progress with that sublime patriotic, democratic, and human faith, which, in our days, should be the very foundation of all generous intelligence."

"Let us never fear robbers or murderers. They are dangers from without, petty dangers. Let us fear ourselves. Prejudices are the real robbers; vices are the real murderers. The great dangers lie within ourselves. What matters it if something threatens are head or our purse! Let us think only of that which threatens the soul."

"If there is anything terrible, if there exists a reality which surpasses dreams, it is this: to live, to see the sun, to be in full possession of viral force; to possess health and joy; to laugh valiantly; to rush toward a glory which one sees dazzling in front of one; to feel in ones's breast lounges which breath, a heart which beats, a will which reasons; to speak, think, hope, love; to have a mother, to have a wife, to have children, to have the light - and all at once, in the space of a shout, in less than a minute, to sink into an abyss; to fall, to roll, to crush, to be crushed, to see ears of wheat, flowers, leaves, branches; not to be able to catch hold of anything; to feel one's sword useless, men beneath one, horses on top of one; to struggle in vain, since ones bones have been broken by some kick in the darkness; to feel a heel which makes ones's eyes start from their sockets; to bite horses' shoes in one's rage,; to stifle. to yell, to writhe; to be beneath, and to say to one's self, "But just a little while ago I was a living man!"

Edward Lear

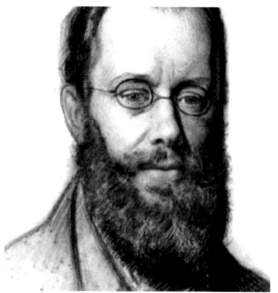

Edward Lear, Public Domain

Edward Lear (1812-1888) Was an English author, musician, poet, and artist who wrote in his *Book of Nonsense* about a duchess with a penchant for farting during dinner parties for the cream of society.

After delivering a gigantic fart that demanded everyone's attention, she turned her icy glare to her stoic butler standing behind here. "Hawkins, stop that" she cried out loud. To which he replied, "Certainly, Your Grace. Which way did it go?"

Famous Quotation:

"How pleasant to know Mr Lear!"
Who has written such volumes of stuff!
Some think him ill-tempered and queer
But a few think him pleasant enough."

Charles Pierre Baudelaire

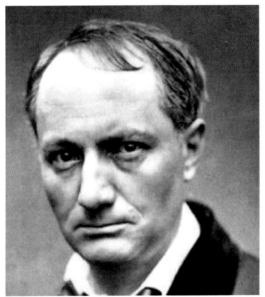

Portrait of Charles Baudelaire, Public Domain

Charles Pierre Baudelaire (1821 – 1867) was a French poet and author who wrote in an original form of prose poetry. He was quoted on the matter of farts:

"Qui s'excuse, s'accuse."

Crepitus was described as the Roman god of flatulence but probably was a fiction created to denigrate Roman theology. He appears as a god in several works of French literature by Voltaire, Charles Baudelaire, and Gustave Flaubert as well as material promoting Roman Catholicism as the true faith.

Famous Quotations:

"The beautiful is always bizarre."

"To handle a language skillfully is to practice a kind of evocative sorcery."

Gustave Flaubert

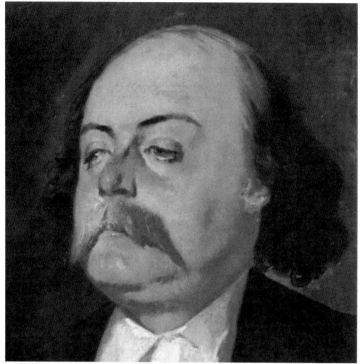

Gustave Flaubert, Public Domain

Gustave Flaubert (1821 – 1880) was a French author whose most famous work is *Madame Bovary*. In his colorful biography he describes his arrival in Jerusalem. "We went in through the Jaffa Gate and I dropped a fart there as I crossed the threshold, quite involuntarily; I was even rather angered by the Voltaireanism of my anus."

Crepitus was described as the Roman god of flatulence but probably was a fiction created to denigrate Roman theology. He appears as a god in several works of French literature by Voltaire, Charles Baudelaire, and Gustave Flaubert as well as material promoting Roman Catholicism as the true faith.

Famous Quotations:

"How wonderful to find in living creatures the same substance as those which make up minerals. Nevertheless they felt a sort of humiliation at the idea that their persons contained phosphorous like matches, albumen like white of egg, hydrogen gas like street lamps."
"Nothing is more humiliating than to see idiots succeed in enterprises we have failed in."

"Travel makes one modest. You see what a tiny place you occupy in the world."
"Do not read, as children do, to amuse yourself, or like the ambitious, for the purpose of instruction. No, read in order to live."
"Be steady and well-ordered in your life so that you can be fierce and original in your work."
"There is not a particle of life which does not bear poetry within it"
"One can be the master of what one does, but never of what one feels."
"The art of writing is the art of discovering what you believe."
"I am irritated by my own writing. I am like a violinist whose ear is true, but whose fingers refuse to reproduce precisely the sound he hears within."
"What better occupation, really, than to spend the evening at the fireside with a book, with the wind beating on the windows and the lamp burning bright...Haven't you ever happened to come across in a book some vague notion that you've had, some obscure idea that returns from afar and that seems to express completely your most subtle feelings?"
"It is always sad to leave a place to which one knows one will never return. Such are the melancolies du voyage: perhaps they are one of the most rewarding things about traveling."
"Pleasure is found first in anticipation, later in memory."
"There is no truth. There is only perception."
"The public wants work which flatters its illusions."
"Sadness is a vice."
"Of all the icy blasts that blow on love, a request for money is the most chilling."
"The most glorious moments in your life are not the so-called days of success, but rather those days when out of dejection and despair you feel rise in you a challenge to life, and the promise of future accomplishments."
"Love art. Of all lies, it is the least untrue."
"Anything becomes interesting if you look at it long enough."
"Thought is the greatest of pleasures —pleasure itself is only imagination—have you ever enjoyed anything more than your dreams?"
"Sentences must stir in a book like leaves in a forest, each distinct from each despite their resemblance."

"God is in the details."
"I have always tried to live in an ivory tower, but a tide of shit is beating at its walls, threatening to undermine it."
"One's duty is to feel what is great, cherish the beautiful, and not accept all the conventions of society with the ignominy that it imposes upon us."
"I have come to have the firm conviction that vanity is the basis of everything."
"By dint of railing at idiots, one runs the risk of becoming an idiot oneself."
"Writing history is like drinking an ocean and pissing a cupful."
"It is a delicious thing to write, whether well or badly - to be no longer yourself but to move in an entire universe of your own creating."
"What vast funds of indifference society possesses"
"In every parting there comes a moment when the beloved is already no longer with us."

"One mustn't look at the abyss, because there is at the bottom an inexpressible charm which attracts us."
"Beautiful things spoil nothing."
"There is always after the death of anyone a kind of stupefaction; so difficult is it to grasp this advent of nothingness and to resign ourselves to believe in it."

Samuel Clemens (Mark Twain)

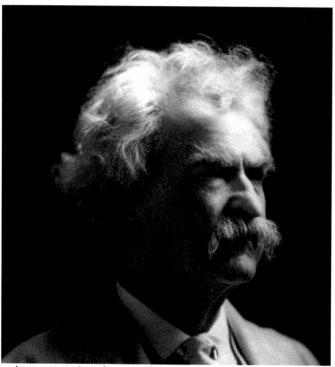

Mark Twain photo portrait. One of a series of photographs taken by A.F. Bradley for the purpose, arranged by George Wharton James, of helping California poet laureate Ina Coolbrith after she lost her home in the fire following the 1906 San Francisco earthquake. In his New York City studio, Bradley placed Twain on a revolving platform to make the capture of different lighting "looks" easier on the subject. The portraits were signed by Twain and sold for Coolbrith's benefit. Twain said four of the series were the finest images ever taken of him. Public Domain

Samuel Langhorne Clemens (1835 -1910), under the pen name Mark Twain, was one of America's most famous authors and humorists. One of his pithy sayings was "Be careful about getting medical advice from a health book, you may die of a misprint." One of his references to farting is in his essay *On Masturbation*. His separate short story *1601* is a more extensive work on the subject.

On Masturbation

"Of all the various kinds of sexual intercourse, this has the least to recommend it. As an amusement, it is too fleeting; as an occupation, it is too wearing; as a public exhibition, there is no money in it. It is unsuited to the drawing room, and in the most cultured society it has long been banished from the social board. It has at last, in our day of progress and improvement, been degraded to brotherhood with flatulence. Among the best bred, these two arts are now indulged in only private -- though by consent of the whole company, when only males are present, it is still permissible, in good society, to remove the embargo on the fundamental sigh."

He wrote a ribald essay entitled *1601* dealing with flatulence in the court of Queen Elizabeth 1. Originally he shared it only with his minister, who encouraged him to publish it to a wider audience. It is reprinted below:

THE FIRST PRINTING Verbatim Reprint [Date, 1601.]
CONVERSATION, AS IT WAS BY THE SOCIAL FIRESIDE, IN THE TIME OF THE TUDORS.

[Mem.--The following is supposed to be an extract from the diary of the Pepys of that day, the same being Queen Elizabeth's cup-bearer. He is supposed to be of ancient and noble lineage; that he despises these literary canaille; that his soul consumes with wrath, to see the queen stooping to talk with such; and that the old man feels that his nobility is defiled by contact with Shakespeare, etc., and yet he has got to stay there till her Majesty chooses to dismiss him.]

YESTERNIGHT toke her maiste ye queene a fantasie such as she sometimes hath, and had to her closet certain that doe write playes, bokes, and such like, these being my lord Bacon, his worship Sir Walter Ralegh, Mr. Ben Jonson, and ye child Francis Beaumonte, which being but sixteen, hath yet turned his hand to ye doing of ye Lattin masters into our Englishe tong, with grete discretion and much applaus.

Also came with these ye famous Shaxpur. A righte straunge mixing truly of mighty blode with mean, ye more in especial since ye queenes grace was present, as likewise these following, to wit: Ye Duchess of Bilgewater, twenty-two yeres of age; ye Countesse of Granby, twenty-six; her doter, ye Lady Helen, fifteen; as also these two maides of honor, to-wit, ye Lady Margery Boothy, sixty-five, and ye Lady Alice Dilberry, turned seventy, she being two yeres ye queenes graces elder.

I being her maites cup-bearer, had no choice but to remaine and beholde rank forgot, and ye high holde converse whye low as uppon equal termes, a grete scandal did ye world heare thereof.
In ye heat of ye talk it befel yt one did breake wind, yielding an exceding mightie and distresfull stink, whereat all did laugh full sore, and then—

Ye Queene.--Verily in mine eight and sixty yeres have I not heard the fellow to this fart. Meseemeth, by ye grete sound and clamour of it, it was male; yet ye belly it did lurk behinde shoulde now fall lean and flat against ye spine of him yt hath bene delivered of so stately and so waste a bulk, where as ye guts of them yt doe quiff-splitters bear, stand comely still and rounde. Prithee let ye author confess ye offspring. Will my Lady Alice testify?

Lady Alice.--Good your grace, an' I had room for such a thundergust within mine ancient bowels, 'tis not in reason I coulde discharge ye same and live to thank God for yt He did choose handmaid so humble whereby to shew his power. Nay, 'tis not I yt have broughte forth this rich o'ermastering fog, this fragrant gloom, so pray you seeke ye further.

Ye Queene.--Mayhap ye Lady Margery hath done ye companie this favor?

Lady Margery.--So please you madam, my limbs are feeble whye weighte and drouth of five and sixty winters, and it behoveth yt I be tender unto them. In ye good providence of God, an' I had contained this wonder, forsoothe wolde I have gi'en 'ye whole evening of my sinking life to ye dribbling of it forth, with trembling and uneasy soul, not launched it sudden in its matchless might, taking mine own life with violence, rending my weak frame like rotten rags. It was not I, your maisty.

Ye Queene.--O' God's name, who hath favored us? Hath it come to pass yt a fart shall fart itself? Not such a one as this, I trow. Young Master Beaumont--but no; 'twould have wafted him to heaven like down of goose's boddy. 'Twas not ye little Lady Helen--nay, ne'er blush, my child; thoul't tickle thy tender maidenhedde with many a mousie-squeak before thou learnest to blow a harricane like this. Wasn't you, my learned and ingenious Jonson?

Jonson.--So fell a blast hath ne'er mine ears saluted, nor yet a stench s o all-pervading and immortal. 'Twas not a novice did it, good your maisty, but one of veteran experience--else hadde he failed of confidence. In sooth it was not I.

Ye Queene.--My lord Bacon?

Lord Bacon.-Not from my leane entrailes hath this prodigy burst forth, so please your grace. Naught doth so befit ye grete as grete performance; and haply shall ye finde yt 'tis not from mediocrity this miracle hath issued.

[Tho' ye subjoct be but a fart, yet will this tedious sink of learning pondrously phillosophize. Meantime did the foul and deadly stink pervade all places to that degree, yt never smelt I ye like, yet dare I not to leave ye presence, albeit I was like to suffocate.]

Ye Queene.--What saith ye worshipful Master Shaxpur?

Shaxpur.--In the great hand of God I stand and so proclaim mine innocence. Though ye sinless hosts of heaven had foretold ye coming of this most desolating breath, proclaiming it a work of uninspired man, its quaking thunders, its firmament-clogging rottenness his own achievement in due course of nature, yet had not I believed it; but had said the pit itself hath furnished forth the stink, and heaven's artillery hath shook the globe in admiration of it.

[Then was there a silence, and each did turn him toward the worshipful Sr Walter Ralegh, that browned, embattled, bloody swashbuckler, who rising up did smile, and simpering say,]

Sr W.--Most gracious maisty, 'twas I that did it, but indeed it was so poor and frail a note, compared with such as I am wont to furnish, yt in sooth I was ashamed to call the weakling mine in so august a presence. It was nothing--less than nothing, madam--I did it but to clear my nether throat; but had I come prepared, then had I delivered something worthy. Bear with me, please your grace, till I can make amends.

[Then delivered he himself of such a godless and rock-shivering blast that all were fain to stop their ears, and following it did come so dense and foul a stink that that which went before did seem a poor and trifling thing beside it. Then saith he, feigning that he blushed and was confused, I perceive that I am weak to-day, and cannot justice do unto my powers; and sat him down as who should say, There, it is not much yet he that hath an arse to spare, let him fellow that, an' he think he can. By God, an' I were ye queene, I would e'en tip this swaggering braggart out o' the court, and let him air his grandeurs and break his intolerable wind before ye deaf and such as suffocation pleaseth.]

Then fell they to talk about ye manners and customs of many peoples, and Master Shaxpur spake of ye boke of ye sieur Michael de Montaine, wherein was mention of ye custom of widows of Perigord to wear uppon ye headdress, in sign of widowhood, a jewel in ye similitude of a man's member wilted and limber, whereat ye queene did laugh and say widows in England doe wear prickes too, but betwixt the thighs, and not wilted neither, till coition hath done that office for them.

Master Shaxpur did likewise observe how yt ye sieur de Montaine hath also spoken of a certain emperor of such mighty prowess that he did take ten maidenheddes in ye compass of a single night, ye while his empress did entertain two and twenty lusty knights between her sheetes, yet was not satisfied; whereat ye merrie Countess Granby saith a ram is yet ye emperor's superior, sith he wil tup above a hundred yewes 'twixt sun and sun; and after, if he can have none more to shag, will masturbate until he hath enrich'd whole acres with his seed.

Then spake ye damned windmill, Sr Walter, of a people in ye uttermost parts of America, yt capulate not until they be five and thirty yeres of age, ye women being eight and twenty, and do it then but once in seven yeres.

Ye Queene.--How doth that like my little Lady Helen? Shall we send thee thither and preserve thy belly?

Lady Helen.--Please your highnesses grace, mine old nurse hath told me there are more ways of serving God than by locking the thighs together; yet am I willing to serve him yt way too, sith your highnesses grace hath set ye ensample.

Ye Queene.--God' wowndes a good answer, childe.

Lady Alice.--Mayhap 'twill weaken when ye hair sprouts below ye navel.

Lady Helen.--Nay, it sprouted two yeres syne; I can scarce more than cover it with my hand now.

Ye Queene.--Hear Ye that, my little Beaumonte? Have ye not a little birde about ye that stirs at hearing tell of so sweete a neste?

Beaumonte.--'Tis not insensible, illustrious madam; but mousing owls and bats of low degree may not aspire to bliss so whelming and ecstatic as is found in ye downy nests of birdes of Paradise.

Ye Queene.--By ye gullet of God, 'tis a neat-turned compliment. With such a tongue as thine, lad, thou'lt spread the ivory thighs of many a willing maide in thy good time, an' thy cod-piece be as handy as thy speeche.

Then spake ye queene of how she met old Rabelais when she was turned of fifteen, and he did tell her of a man his father knew that had a double pair of bollocks, whereon a controversy followed as concerning the most just way to spell the word, ye contention running high betwixt ye learned Bacon and ye ingenious Jonson, until at last ye old Lady Margery, wearying of it all, saith, 'Gentles, what mattereth it how ye shall spell the word?

I warrant Ye when ye use your bollocks ye shall not think of it; and my Lady Granby, be ye content; let the spelling be, ye shall enjoy the beating of them on your buttocks just the same, I trow. Before I had gained my fourteenth year I had learnt that them that would explore a cunt stop'd not to consider the spelling o't.'

Sr W.--In sooth, when a shift's turned up, delay is meet for naught but dalliance. Boccaccio hath a story of a priest that did beguile a maid into his cell, then knelt him in a corner to pray for grace to be rightly thankful for this tender maidenhead ye Lord had sent him; but ye abbot, spying through ye key-hole, did see a tuft of brownish hair with fair white flesh about it, wherefore when ye priest's prayer was done, his chance was gone, forasmuch as ye little maid had but ye one cunt, and that was already occupied to her content.

Then conversed they of religion, and ye mightie work ye old dead Luther did doe by ye grace of God. Then next about poetry, and Master Shaxpur did rede a part of his King Henry IV. Ye which, it seemeth unto me, is not of ye value of an arsefull of ashes, yet they praised it bravely, one and all.

Ye same did rede a portion of his "Venus and Adonis," to their prodigious admiration, whereas I, being sleepy and fatigued withal, did deme it but paltry stuff, and was the more discomforted in that ye blody bucanier had got his wind again, and did turn his mind to farting with such villain zeal that presently I was like to choke once more. God damn this windy ruffian and all his breed. I wolde that hell mighte get him.

They talked about ye wonderful defense which old Sr. Nicholas Throgmorton did make for himself before ye judges in ye time of Mary; which was unlucky matter to broach, sith it fetched out ye quene with a 'Pity ythe, having so much wit, had yet not enough to save his doter's maidenhedde sound for her marriage-bed.' And ye quene did give ye damn'd Sr. Walter a look yt made hym wince--for she hath not forgot he was her own lover it yt olde day.

There was silent uncomfortableness now; 'twas not a good turn for talk to take, sith if ye queene must find offense in a little harmless debauching, when pricks were stiff and cunts not loathe to take ye stiffness out of them, who of this company was sinless; behold, was not ye wife of Master Shaxpur four months gone with child when she stood uppe before ye altar?

Was not her Grace of Bilgewater roger'd by four lords before she had a husband? Was not ye little Lady Helen born on her mother's wedding-day? And, beholde, were not ye Lady Alice and ye Lady Margery there, mouthing religion, whores from ye cradle?

In time came they to discourse of Cervantes, and of the new painter, Rubens, that is beginning to be heard of. Fine words and dainty-wrought phrases from the ladies now, one or two of them being, in other days, pupils of that poor ass, Lille, himself; and I marked how that Jonson and Shaxpur did fidget to discharge some venom of sarcasm, yet dared they not in the presence, the queene's grace being ye very flower of ye Euphuists herself.

But behold, these be they yt, having a specialty, and admiring it in themselves, be jealous when a neighbor doth essaye it, nor can abide it in them long. Wherefore 'twas observable yt ye quene waxed uncontent; and in time labor'd grandiose speeche out of ye mouth of Lady Alice, who manifestly did mightily pride herself thereon, did quite exhauste ye quene's endurance, who listened till ye gaudy speeche was done, then lifted up her brows, and with vaste irony, mincing saith 'O shit!' Whereat they alle did laffe, but not ye Lady Alice, yt olde foolish bitche.

Now was Sr. Walter minded of a tale he once did hear ye ingenious Margrette of Navarre relate, about a maid, which being like to suffer rape by an olde archbishoppe, did smartly contrive a device to save her maidenhedde, and said to him, First, my lord, I prithee, take out thy holy tool and piss before me; which doing, lo his member felle, and would not rise again.

Famous Quotations:

"If you tell the truth, you don't have to remember anything."
"Whenever you find yourself on the side of the majority, it is time to pause and reflect."
 "The man who does not read has no advantage over the man who cannot read."
"Never put off till tomorrow what may be done day after tomorrow just as well".
"I have never let my schooling interfere with my education."
"Classic' - a book which people praise and don't read."
"A lie can travel half way around the world while the truth is putting on its shoes."
"Never tell the truth to people who are not worthy of it."
"The fear of death follows from the fear of life. A man who lives fully is prepared to die at any time."
"Be careful about reading health books. You may die of a misprint."
"Keep away from people who try to belittle your ambitions. Small people always do that, but the really great make you feel that you, too, can become great."
"In a good bookroom you feel in some mysterious way that you are absorbing the wisdom contained in all the books through your skin, without even opening them."
"Reader, suppose you were an idiot. And suppose you were a member of Congress. But I repeat myself."
 "Don't go around saying the world owes you a living. The world owes you nothing. It was here first."
"God created war so that Americans would learn geography."
"I did not attend his funeral, but I sent a nice letter saying I approved of it."
 "Life is short, Break the Rules.
Forgive quickly, Kiss SLOWLY.
Love truly. Laugh uncontrollably
And never regret ANYTHING
That makes you smile."
"The difference between the right word and the almost right word is the difference between lightning and a lightning bug."
"Loyalty to country ALWAYS. Loyalty to government, when it deserves it."
"Never allow someone to be your priority while allowing yourself to be their option."
"Wrinkles should merely indicate where the smiles have been."
"Truth is stranger than fiction, but it is because Fiction is obliged to stick to possibilities; Truth isn't."
"Books are for people who wish they were somewhere else."
"What would men be without women? Scarce, sir...mighty scarce."
"I do not fear death. I had been dead for billions and billions of years before I was born, and had not suffered the slightest inconvenience from it."
"Clothes make the man. Naked people have little or no influence on society."

"Don't part with your illusions. When they are gone you may still exist, but you have ceased to live."

"Always do what is right. It will gratify half of mankind and astound the other."

"If you pick up a starving dog and make him prosperous he will not bite you. This is the principal difference between a dog and man."

"You can't depend on your eyes when your imagination is out of focus."

"When I was a boy of 14, my father was so ignorant I could hardly stand to have the old man around. But when I got to be 21, I was astonished at how much the old man had learned in seven years."

"The trouble is not in dying for a friend, but in finding a friend worth dying for."

"If you don't read the newspaper, you're uninformed. If you read the newspaper, you're mis-informed."

"Courage is resistance to fear, mastery of fear - not absence of fear."

"It's not the size of the dog in the fight, it's the size of the fight in the dog."

"Travel is fatal to prejudice, bigotry, and narrow-mindedness, and many of our people need it sorely on these accounts. Broad, wholesome, charitable views of men and things cannot be acquired by vegetating in one little corner of the earth all one's lifetime."

"Name the greatest of all inventors. Accident."

"Kindness is a language which the deaf can hear and the blind can see."

"I've lived through some terrible things in my life, some of which actually happened."

"Everyone is a moon, and has a dark side which he never shows to anybody."

"The best way to cheer yourself is to try to cheer someone else up."

"The easy confidence with which I know another man's religion is folly teaches me to suspect that my own is also."

"Education: the path from cocky ignorance to miserable uncertainty."

"The secret to getting ahead is getting started."

"All you need in this life is ignorance and confidence; then success is sure. "

"Get your facts first, and then you can distort them as much as you please."

"A clear conscience is the sure sign of a bad memory."

"History doesn't repeat itself, but it does rhyme."

"A banker is a fellow who lends you his umbrella when the sun is shining, but wants it back the minute it begins to rain."

"April 1. This is the day upon which we are reminded of what we are on the other three hundred and sixty-four."

"Forgiveness is the fragrance that the violet sheds on the heel that has crushed it."

"Out of all the things I have lost, I miss my mind the most."

"I didn't have time to write a short letter, so I wrote a long one instead."

"I must have a prodigious amount of mind; it takes me as much as a week, sometimes, to make it up!"

"Any emotion, if it is sincere, is involuntary."

"When angry, count four. When very angry, swear."

"Of all the animals, man is the only one that is cruel. He is the only one that inflicts pain for the pleasure of doing it."

"The most interesting information come from children, for they tell all they know and then stop."

"I have found out that there ain't no surer way to find out whether you like people or hate them than to travel with them."

"To get the full value of joy you must have someone to divide it with."

"When we remember we are all mad, the mysteries disappear and life stands explained."

"The human race has only one really effective weapon and that is laughter."

"It is curious that physical courage should be so common in the world and moral courage so rare."

"Always acknowledge a fault. This will throw those in authority off their guard and give you an opportunity to commit more."

"The two most important days in your life are the day you are born and the day you find out why."

"Anger is an acid that can do more harm to the vessel in which it is stored than to anything on which it is poured."

"Giving up smoking is the easiest thing in the world. I know because I've done it thousands of times."

"Never argue with stupid people, they will drag you down to their level and then beat you with experience."

"There is a charm about the forbidden that makes it unspeakably desirable."

"Part of the secret of success in life is to eat what you like and let the food fight it out inside."

"It is better to deserve honors and not have them than to have them and not deserve them."

"Education consists mainly of what we have unlearned."

"There are many humorous things in the world; among them, the white man's notion that he is less savage than the other savages."

"My books are water; those of the great geniuses is wine. Everybody drinks water."

"There was never yet an uninteresting life. Such a thing is an impossibility. Inside of the dullest exterior there is a drama, a comedy, and a tragedy."

"Reality can be beaten with enough imagination."

"It takes your enemy and your friend, working together, to hurt you to the heart: the one to slander you and the other to get the news to you."

"Action speaks louder than words but not nearly as often."

"Obscurty and a competence—that is the life that is best worth living."

"Eat a live frog first thing in the morning and nothing worse will happen to you the rest of the day."

"Man is the only animal that blushes. Or needs to."

"Thunder is good, thunder is impressive; but it is lightening that does the work."

"If Christ were here there is one thing he would not be—a Christian."

"The right word may be effective, but no word was ever as effective as a rightly timed pause."

"I've had a lot of worries in my life, most of which never happened."

"There's one way to find out if a man is honest: ask him; if he says yes, you know he's crooked."

"Few things are harder to put up with than the annoyance of a good example."

"A half-truth is the most cowardly of lies."

"In the first place God made idiots. This was for practice. Then he made school boards."

"Let us be thankful for the fools. But for them the rest of us could not succeed. "

"When you fish for love, bait with your heart, not your brain."

"Why do you sit there looking like an envelope without any address on it?"

"Let us live so that when we come to die even the undertaker will be sorry."

"It's better to keep your mouth shut and appear stupid than open it and remove all doubt"

"I thoroughly disapprove of duels. If a man should challenge me, I would take him kindly and forgivingly by the hand and lead him to a quiet place and kill him."

"If voting made any difference they wouldn't let us do it."

"Just because you're taught that something's right and everyone believes it's right, it don't make it right."

"Life does not consist mainly, or even largely, of facts or happenings. It consist mainly of the storm of thoughts that is forever flowing through one's head."

"Often it does seem such a pity that Noah and his party did not miss the boat."

"Under certain circumstances, profanity provides a relief denied even to prayer."

"The reports of my death are greatly exaggerated."

"Be good and you will be lonesome."

"Writing is easy. All you have to do is cross out the wrong words."

"A successful book is not made of what is in it, but what is left out of it."

"Noise proves nothing. Often a hen who has laid an egg cackles as if she had laid an asteroid."

"A man cannot be comfortable without his own approval."

"It is by the goodness of god that in our country we have those 3 unspeakably precious things: freedom of speech, freedom of conscience, and the prudence never to practice either of them."

"Don't wake up a woman in love. Let her dream, so that she does not weep when she returns to her bitter reality"

"Worrying is like paying a debt you don't owe."

"Patriotism is supporting your country all the time and your government when it deserves it."

"The fact that man knows right from wrong proves his intellectual superiority to the other creatures; but the fact that he can do wrong proves his moral inferiority to any creatures that cannot."

"The man who is a pessimist before 48 knows too much; if he is an optimist after it he knows too little."

"Humor is mankind's greatest blessing."

"He who asks is a fool for five minutes, but he who does not ask remains a fool forever."

"That is just the way with some people. They get down on a thing when they don't know nothing about it."

"I can teach anybody how to get what they want out of life. The problem is that I

can't find anybody who can tell me what they want."
"The lack of money is the root of all evil."
"Too much of anything is bad, but too much good whiskey is barely enough."
"It's easier to fool people than to convince them that they have been fooled."
"Civilization is a limitless multiplication of unnecessary necessaries."
"Familiarity breeds contempt and children."
"Let us consider that we are all partially insane. It will explain us to each other; it will unriddle many riddles; it will make clear and simple many things which are involved in haunting and harassing difficulties and obscurities now."
"Grief can take care of itself, but to get the full value of joy you must have somebody to divide it with."
"Never argue with a fool, onlookers may not be able to tell the difference."
"The older I get, the more clearly I remember things that never happened."
"It's easy to make friends, but hard to get rid of them."
"No man's life, liberty, or property are safe while the legislature is in session."
"Censorship is telling a man he can't have a steak just because a baby can't chew it."
"Facts are stubborn things, but statistics are pliable."
"Politicians and diapers must be changed often, and for the same reason."
"There is nothing so annoying as having two people talking when you're busy interrupting."
"It usually takes me two or three days to prepare an impromptu speech."
"The more I learn about people, the more I like my dog."
"Distance lends enchantment to the view."
"Be respectful to your superiors, if you have any."
"great people are those who make others feel that they, too, can become great."
"The secret of getting ahead is getting started. The secret of getting started is breaking your complex overwhelming tasks into small manageable tasks, and starting on the first one."
"for business reasons, I must preserve the outward signs of sanity."
"I take my only exercise acting as a pallbearer at the funerals of my friends who exercise regularly."
"The radical of one century is the conservative of the next. The radical invents the views. When he has worn them out, the conservative adopt."
"Travel is fatal to prejudice, bigotry, and narrow-mindedness."
"Do something everyday that you don't want to do; this is the golden rule for acquiring the habit of doing your duty without pain."
"Good judgment is the result of experience and experience the result of bad judgment."
"It could probably be shown by facts and figures that there is no distinctly native American criminal class except Congress."
"There is no sadder sight than a young pessimist, except an old optimist."
"In Paris they just simply opened their eyes and stared when we spoke to them in French! We never did succeed in making those idiots understand their own language."
"A man is accepted into a church for what he believes and he is turned out for

what he knows."

"Religion was invented when the first con man met the first fool."

"Whiskey is for drinking; water is for fighting over."

"It is easier to stay out than to get out."

"The secret source of humor is not joy but sorrow; there is no humor in heaven."

"Against the assault of laughter, nothing can stand."

"Comparison is the death of joy."

"Honesty: The best of all the lost arts."

"A man is never more truthful than when he acknowledges himself a liar."

"There are three things men can do with women: love them, suffer them, or turn them into literature."

"There are several good protections against temptations, but the surest is cowardice."

"The only difference between a tax man and a taxidermist is that the taxidermist leaves the skin."

"Age is an issue of mind over matter. If you don't mind, it doesn't matter."

"I can last two months on a good compliment."

"I always take Scotch whiskey at night as a preventive of toothache. I have never had the toothache; and what is more, I never intend to have it."

"If books are not good company, where shall I find it?"

"To do good is noble. To tell others to do good is even nobler and much less trouble."

"Explaining humor is a lot like dissecting a frog, you learn a lot in the process, but in the end you kill it."

"December is the toughest month of the year. Others are July, January, September, April, November, May, March, June, October, August, and February."

"Man was made at the end of the week's work when God was tired."

"The less there is to justify a traditional custom, the harder it is to get rid of it"

"Plain question and plain answer make the shortest road out of most perplexities."

"Most writers regard the truth as their most valuable possession, and therefore are economical in its use."

"New Orleans food is as delicious as the less criminal forms of sin."

"Every person is a book, each year a chapter,"

"I couldn't bear to think about it; and yet, somehow, I couldn't think about nothing else."

"When in doubt tell the truth. It will confound your enemies and astound your friends."

"One of the most striking differences between a cat and a lie is that a cat has only nine lives."

"Habit is habit, and not to be flung out of the window by any man, but coaxed down-stairs one step at a time."

"Conservatism is the blind and fear-filled worship of dead radicals."

"I wish I could make him understand that a loving good heart is riches enough, and that without it intellect is poverty."

"If we would learn what the human race really is at bottom, we need only observe it in election times."

"He had had much experience of physicians, and said 'the only way to keep your health is to eat what you don't want, drink what you don't like, and do what you'd druther not'."

"Education: that which reveals to the wise, and conceals from the stupid, the vast limits of their knowledge."

"I was sorry to have my name mentioned as one of the great authors, because they have a sad habit of dying off. Chaucer is dead, Spencer is dead, so is Milton, so is Shakespeare, and I'm not feeling so well myself."

"Nothing that grieves us can be called little: by the eternal laws of proportion a child's loss of a doll and a king's loss of a crown are events of the same size."

"Never be haughty to the humble, never be humble to the haughty."

"Good breeding consists of concealing how much we think of ourselves and how little we think of the other person."

"It's not what you don't know that kills you, it's what you know for sure that ain't true."

"Anyone who can only think of one way to spell a word obviously lacks imagination."

"She remained both girl and woman to the last day of her life. Under a grave and gentle exterior burned inextinguishable fires of sympathy, energy, devotion, enthusiasm, and absolutely limitless affection."

"We should be careful to get out of an experience only the wisdom that is in it and stop there lest we be like the cat that sits down on a hot stove lid. She will never sit down on a hot stove lid again and that is well but also she will never sit down on a cold one anymore."

"Let us not be too particular. It is better to have old second-hand diamonds than none at all."

"The only difference between reality and fiction is that fiction needs to be credible."

"You can't reason with your heart; it has its own laws, and thumps about things which the intellect scorns."

"Peace by persuasion has a pleasant sound, but I think we should not be able to work it. We should have to tame the human race first, and history seems to show that that cannot be done."

"High and fine literature is wine, and mine is only water; but everybody likes water."

"All I care to know about a man is that he is a human being... he can't be any worse."

"Most people are bothered by those passages of Scripture they do not understand, but the passages that bother me are those I do understand."

"The difference between a Miracle and a Fact is exactly the difference between a mermaid and a seal."

"Just when I thought I was learning how to live, 'twas then I realized I was learning how to die."

"If everyone was satisfied with himself, there would be no heroes."

"the more I know about people, the better I like my dogs."

"Loyalty to a petrified opinion never yet broke a chain or freed a human soul."

"Be careless in your dress if you must, but keep a tidy soul."

"The holy passion of Friendship is of so sweet and steady and loyal and enduring a nature that it will last through a whole lifetime, if not asked to lend money."

"I do not wish any reward but to know I have done the right thing."

"I do not like work even when someone else is doing it."

"The more things are forbidden, the more popular they become."

"Nature knows no indecencies; man invents them."

"Man - a figment of God's imagination."

"Human pride is not worthwhile; there is always something lying in wait to take the wind out of it."

"There are some few people I respect and admire, but I don't think much of the species."

"Focus more on your desire than on your doubt, and the dream will take care of itself."

"Nothing so needs reforming as other people's habits."

"How little a thing can make us happy when we feel that we have earned it."

"Drawing on my fine command of language, I said nothing."

"If people are good only because they fear punishment, and hope for reward, then we are a sorry lot indeed."

"One frequently only finds out how really beautiful a women is, until after considerable acquaintance with her."

"Give every day the chance to become the most beautiful day of your life."

"Wit is the sudden marriage of ideas which before their union were not perceived to have any relation. "

"There is something fascinating about science. One gets such wholesale returns of conjecture out of such a trifling investment of fact."

"Why not go out on a limb? That's where the fruit is."

"I am a great and sublime fool. But then I am God's fool, and all His works must be contemplated with respect."

"One should never use exclamation points in writing. It is like laughing at your own joke."

"Give a man a reputation as an early riser and he can sleep 'til noon."

"That's the difference between governments and individuals. Governments don't care, individuals do."

"Necessity is the mother of taking chances."

"Humor is the great thing, the saving thing. The minute it crops up, all our irritations and resentments slip away and a sunny spirit takes their place."

"What work I have done I have done because it has been play. If it had been work I shouldn't have done it. . . . The work that is really a man's own work is play and not work at all. . . . When we talk about the great workers of the world we really mean the great players of the world."

"The rule is perfect: in all matters of opinion our adversaries are insane."

"Wagner's music is better than it sounds."

"Stars and shadows ain't good to see by."

"By trying we can easily learn to endure adversity – another man's, I mean."

"An honest politician is an oxymoron."

"A person with a new idea is a crank until the idea succeeds."

"The trouble with the world is not that people know too little; it's that they know so many things that just aren't so. "

"Really great people make you feel that you, too, can become great."

"It is higher and nobler to be kind."

"I cannot call to mind a single instance where I have ever been irreverent, except toward the things which were sacred to other people."

"I don't like to commit myself about Heaven and Hell, you see, I have friends in both places."

"Love is not a product of reasonings and statistics. It just comes -none knows whence-and cannot explain itself."

"I don't want no better book than what your face is."

"Never have a battle of wits with an unarmed person."

"I was born lazy. I am no lazier now than I was forty years ago, but that is because I reached the limit forty years ago. You can't go beyond possibility."

"Don't let schooling interfere with your education."

"Everything has its limit - iron ore cannot be educated into gold."

"I have been complimented many times and they always embarrass me; I always feel they have not said enough."

"I wonder if God created man because He was disappointed with the monkey."

"You meet people who forget you. You forget people you meet. But sometimes you meet those people you can't forget. Those are your 'friends"

"The human race is a race of cowards; and I am not only marching in that procession but carrying a banner."

"Now he found out a new thing--namely, that to promise not to do a thing is the surest way in the world to make a body want to go and do that very thing."

"Fame is a vapor, popularity an accident; the only earthly certainty is oblivion."

"They did not know it was impossible so they did it"

"Don't go around thinking the world owes you a living. It was here first."

"Whoever is happy will make others happy too."

"Only one thing is impossible for God: To find any sense in any copyright law on the planet."

"If you must be indiscrete, be discrete in your indiscretion."

"Put all your eggs in one basket and then watch that basket."

"If you want me to give you a two-hour presentation, I am ready today. If you want only a five-minute speech, it will take me two weeks to prepare."

"It is just like man's vanity and impertinence to call an animal dumb because it is dumb to his dull perceptions. "

"Why is it that we rejoice at a birth and grieve at a funeral? It is because we are not the person involved."

"If a person offends you, and you are in doubt as to whether it was intentional or not, do not resort to extreme measures; simply watch your chance, and hit him with a brick."

"I have been studying the traits and dispositions of the "lower animals" (so called) and contrasting them with the traits and dispositions of man. I find the result humiliating to me."

"Let us make a special effort to stop communicating with each other, so we can have some conversation."

"Choosing not to read is like closing an open door to paradise"

"Broad, wholesome, charitable views of men and things can not be acquired by vegetating in one little corner of the earth all one's lifetime."

"When majority is insane, sane must go to asylum."

"I am not one of those who in expressing opinions confine themselves to facts."

"We have a criminal jury system which is superior to any in the world and it's efficiency is only marred by the difficulty of finding twelve men every day who don't know anything and can't read-"

"The very ink with which all history is written is merely fluid prejudice."

"Work like you don't need the money. Dance like no one is watching. And love like you've never been hurt."

"The history of our race, and each individual's experience, are sown thick with evidence that a truth is not hard to kill and that a lie told well is immortal."

"Learning softeneth the heart and breedeth gentleness and charity."

"There is no such thing as an ordinary life."

"If you don't like the weather in New England now, just wait a few minutes."

"New Year's Day: Now is the accepted time to make your regular annual good resolutions. Next week you can begin paving hell with them as usual."

"There are two times in a man's life when he should not speculate: when he can't afford it, and when he can."

"A discriminating irreverence is the creator and protector of human liberty."

"The pitifulest thing out is a mob; that's what an army is --a mob; they don't fight with courage that's born in them, but with courage that's borrowed from their mass, and from their officers. But a mob without any MAN at the head of it is BENEATH pitifulness."

"To be a patriot, one had to say, and keep on saying, "Our Country, right or wrong," and urge on the little war. Have you not perceived that that phrase is an insult to the nation?"

"The joy of killing! the joy of seeing killing done - these are traits of the human race at large."

"If you don't know how to pronounce a word, say it loudly. Do not compound mispronunciation with inaudibility"

"When ill luck begins, it does not come in sprinkles, but in showers."

"A person who won't read has no advantage over one who can't read."

"Do the thing you fear the most and the death of fear is certain."

"Well, there are times when one would like to hang the whole human race and finish the farce."

"I believe I have no prejudices whatsoever. All I need to know is that a man is a member of the human race. That's bad enough for me."

"October: This is one of the peculiarly dangerous months to speculate in stocks. The others are July, January, September, April, November, May, March, June, December, August and February."

"I am only human, although I regret it."

"How empty is theory in the presence of fact!"

"the size of a misfortune is not determinable by an outsider's measurement of it but only by the measurements applied to it by the person specially affected by it."

"I've never wished a man dead, but I have read some obituaries with great pleasure."

"Golf is a good walk spoiled."

"We have not the reverent feeling for the rainbow that the savage has, because we know how it is made. We have lost as much as we gained by prying into that matter."

"We can't all be heros because someone has to sit on the curb and clap as they go by."

"Everybody lies...every day, every hour, awake, asleep, in his dreams, in his joy, in his mourning. If he keeps his tongue still his hands, his feet, his eyes, his attitude will convey deception."

"Advertisements contain the only truths to be relied on in a newspaper."

"Always read stuff that will make you look good if you die in the middle of it."

"I have been on the verge of being an angel all my life, but it's never happened yet."

"I haven't a particle of confidence in a man who has no redeeming petty vices whatsoever."

"Each place has its own advantages - heaven for the climate, and hell for the society."

"Life would be infinitely happier if we could only be born at the age of eighty and gradually approach eighteen."

"You have heretofore found out, by my teachings, that man is a fool; you are now aware that woman is a damned fool."

"If it's your job to eat a frog, it's best to do it first thing in the morning. And if it's your job to eat two frogs, it's best to eat the biggest one first."

"I am not interested to know whether vivisection produces results that are profitable to the human race or doesn't...The pain which it inflicts upon unconsenting animals is the basis of my enmity toward it, and it is to me sufficient justification of the enmity without looking further."

"a fully belly is little worth where the mind is starved."

"When the Lord finished the world, he pronounced it good. That is what I said about my first work, too. But Time, I tell you, Time takes the confidence out of these incautious opinions. It is more than likely that He thinks about the world, now, pretty much as I think about the Innocents Abroad. The fact is, there is a trifle too much water in both."

"The air up there in the clouds is very pure and fine, bracing and delicious. And why shouldn't it be?--it is the same the angels breathe."

"I have too much respect for the truth to drag it out on every trifling occasion."

"At noon I observed a bevy of nude young native women bathing in the sea, and I went and sat down on there clothes to keep them from being stolen."

"A sound heart is a surer guide than an ill-trained conscience."

"Additional problems are the offspring of poor solutions."

"He was endowed with a stupidity which by the least little stretch would go

around the globe four times and tie."
"It is my belief that nearly any invented quotation, played with confidence, stands a good chance to deceive."
"Let us consider that we are all insane. It will explain us to each other. It will unriddle many riddles"
"Cauliflower is nothing but cabbage with a college education."
"The ability to find solutions to life's challenges is what makes us grow as a person."
"The humorous story is told gravely; the teller does his best to conceal the fact that he even dimly suspects that there is anything funny about it."
"Memories which someday will become all beautiful when the last annoyance that encumbers them shall have faded out of our minds."
"The secret of success is making your vocation your vacation."
"Some people get an education without going to college. The rest get it after they get out."
"Don't explain your author, read him right and he explains himself."
"Eschew surplusage." .
"I do not like an injurious lie, except when it injures somebody else."
"Eloquence is the essential thing in a speech, not information."
"To get the right word in the right place is a rare achievement."
"I cannot see how a man of any large degree of humorous perception can ever be religious -- unless he purposely shut the eyes of his mind & keep them shut by force."
"Sane and intelligent human beings are like all other human beings, and carefully and cautiously and diligently conceal their private real opinions from the world and give out fictitious ones in their stead for general consumption."
"I have never taken any exercise except sleeping and resting."
"A sincere compliment is always grateful to a lady, so long as you don't try to knock her down with it."
"Find a job you enjoy doing, and you will never have to work a day in your life."
"I was seldom able to see an opportunity until it had ceased to be one."
"I was dead for millions of years before I was born and it never inconvenienced me a bit."
"I have been an author for 20 years and an ass for 55."
"My experience of men had long ago taught me that one of the surest ways of begetting an enemy was to do some stranger an act of kindness which should lay upon him the irritating sense of an obligation."
"You cant reach old age by another man's road, my habits protect my life but they would assassinate you"
"We recognize that there are no trivial occurrences in life if we get the right focus on them."
"Cheer up, the worst is yet to come!"
"Continuous improvement is better than delayed perfection."
"There is nothing in the world like persuasive speech to fuddle the mental apparatus."
"Children and fools always speak the truth."

"Don't use a five-dollar word when a fifty-cent word will do."

"Total abstinence is so excellent a thing that it cannot be carried to too great an extent. In my passion for it I even carry it so far as to totally abstain from total abstinence itself."

"The best of all lost arts is honesty"

"A good lawyer knows the law; a clever one takes the judge to lunch."

"Our opinions do not really blossom into fruition until we have expressed them to someone else."

"Work and play are words used to describe the same thing under differing conditions."

"Nothing so needs reforming as other people's habits."

"Man is the only animal that loves his neighbor as himself and cuts his throat if his theology isn't straight"

"The more I the more I know people the more I like my dog"

"Life should begin with age and it's privileges and accumulations, and end with youth and it's capacity to splendidly enjoy such advantages."

"Climate is what we expect, weather is what we get."

"Switzerland would me a mighty big place if it were ironed flat."

"You cannot trust your eyes, if your imagination is out of focus."

"Truth is the most valuable thing we have. Let us economize it."

"Honesty is the best policy - when there is money in it."

"Buy land, they're not making it anymore."

"What a hell of a heaven it will be when they get all these hypocrites assembled there!"

"There are ten parts of speech and they are all troublesome."

"A woman's intuition is better than a man's. Nobody knows anything, really, you know, and a woman can guess a good deal nearer than a man."

"Patriot: the person who can holler the loudest without knowing what he is hollering about."

"The less a man knows the bigger the noise he makes and the higher the salary he commands."

"The difference between nonfiction and fiction is that fiction must be absolutely believable."

"The truth should never be permitted to stand in the way of a good story."

"Denial ain't just a river in Egypt."

"Warm summer sun,
shine brightly here,
Warm Southern wind,
blow softly here,
Green sod above,
lie light, lie light,
Good night, dear heart;
good night, good night."

"Part of the secret of success in life is to eat what you want."

"Concerning the difference between man and the jackass: some observers hold that there isn't any. But this wrongs the jackass."

"In Paris they simply stared at me when I spoke to them in French. I never did succeed in making those idiots understand their language."

"Faith is believing what you know ain't so."

"History may not repeat itself, but it does rhyme a lot."

"If God had meant for us to be naked, we'd have been born that way."

"A little starvation can really do more for the average sick man than can the best of medicines and the best doctors "

"In certain trying circumstances, urgent circumstances, desperate circumstances, profanity furnishes a relief denied even to prayer."

"Many a small thing has been made large by the right kind of advertising."

"Truth is stranger than fiction."

"It is strange the way the ignorant and inexperienced so often and so undeservedly succeed when the informed and the experienced fail. All you need in this life is ignorance and confidence, and then success is sure."

"I have no color prejudices nor caste prejudices nor creed prejudices. All I care to know is that a man is a human being, and that is enough for me; he can't be any worse.."

"I find that the further I go back, the better things were, whether they happened or not."

"Never learn to do anything: if you don't learn, you'll always find someone else to do it for you."

"I am prepared to meet anyone, but whether anyone is prepared for the great ordeal of meeting me is another matter"

"Health is a habit, and not to be flung out of the window by any man, but coaxed downstairs a step at a time."

"Suppose you were an idiot. And suppose you were a member of Congress. But I repeat myself."

"To succeed in life, you need two things: ignorance and confidence."

"A thing long expected takes the form of the unexpected when at last it comes."

"To cease smoking is the easiest thing I ever did. I ought to know because I've done it a thousand times."

"I have made it a rule never to smoke more than one cigar at a time. I have no other restriction as regards smoking."

"Never argue with stupid people, they will drag you down to their level and then beat you with experience"

"I installed a skylight in my apartment... the people who live above me are furious!"

"Beware of health books. You may die of a misprint."

"There are basically two types of people. People who accomplish things, and people who claim to have accomplished things. The first group is less crowded."

"You will be more disappointed in life by the things that you do not do than by the things that you do."

"It takes three weeks to prepare a good ad-lib speech."

"Sing like no one is listening, love like you've never been hurt, dance like nobody is watching, and live like it's heaven on earth."

"Most people use statistics like a drunk man uses a lamppost; more for support than illumination"

"Noise proves nothing. Often a hen who has merely laid an egg cackles as if she has laid an asteroid."

"Do the right thing. It will gratify some people and astonish the rest."

"It is noble to teach oneself, but still nobler to teach others --and less trouble."

"A consciously exaggerated compliment is an offense."

"Everybody talks about the weather, but nobody does anything about it.

"All emotion is involuntary when genuine."

"Life is planned with one principle objective to make you do all the particular things you particularly don't want to do."

No man's life, liberty, and property are safe while the legislature is in session."

"I know all about audiences, they believe everything you say, except when you are telling the truth."

"Civilization is a limitless multiplication of unnecessary necessities"

"Never attribute to malice what can be adequately explained by stupidity."

"In the first place, God made idiots. That was for practice. Then he made school boards."

"Often, the surest way to convey misinformation is to tell the strict truth."

"I sometimes wonder if our world leaders are very smart and just putting us on, or very stupid and mean it."

Émile Zola

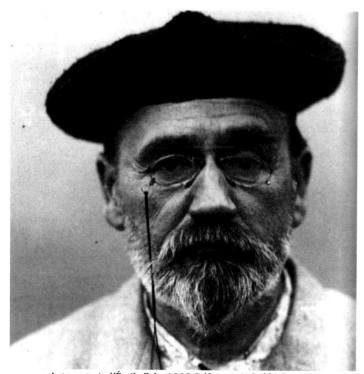

Autoportrait d'Émile Zola. 1902 Self portrait. Public Domain

Émile Édouard Charles Antoine Zola (1840 – 1902) was a French author and journalist. His style known as naturalism described every detail of the human condition, warts and all.

In *La Terre* (the 15th volume of the series Les Rougon-Macquart), the eldest Fouan son (called Jesus Christ because of his long hair and beard) farts at will, and wins free drinks by betting on his extraordinary farting skills.

La Terre:

Jesus Christ was very windy continual blowing winds in the home and stood in joy. No, damn! we are not bothered with the guy because he does not let go one without the support of a farce. He repudiated those timid noises, smothered between two leathers, fusing with Left anxiety; he never had that frank detonations of strength and a cannon of scale; and, each time, the thigh lifted, in a move to ease and swagger, he called his daughter, an urgent voice command, severe air: --The Funk quickly here, dammit!

 She ran, the coup was leaving, was shot in the void, so vibrant, she jumped. -- Cours Later! and passes it between your teeth, to see if there are knots! Other times, when she arrived, he gave her his hand. --Tire Therefore cloth! Let's crack! And as soon as the explosion occurred, with the tumult and bubbling mine too drunk: --Ah! it's hard, thank you all the same! Or put it plays an imaginary gun, aimed at length; then, the gun unloaded: --Va Seek, brings lazy! Slutty suffocated, fell on his back, as she laughed.

This was an ever-changing and growing gaiety she might know the game, expect the final thunder, he still carried in the perennial comic of its turbulence. Oh! the father, was it pretty funny! Sometimes he spoke of a tenant who does not pay his term and that flanked outside; sometimes, he turned in surprise, saluted seriously, as if the table had said hello; sometimes it was a whole bouquet for the Cure for the mayor and for the ladies. One would thought the guy was pulling his belly he wanted a real box music; so that at Bon Laboureur in Cloyes, we bet, "I pay you a glass, if you make it six, "and he was six, he earned all hits. It turned to glory, Funk was proud, amused, if twisting in advance, as soon as he raised his thigh, constantly admiration before him in terror and tenderness he inspired.

And in the evening installing the father Fouan the castle, as it was known the old cellar where the poacher was hiding from the first meal that daughter served to his father and his grandfather standing behind them respectful servant, cheerfulness and rang, very high. The old man had given franc, smell good spread, red beans and veal with onions, cook the little licking fingers. Such As she brought the beans, she almost broke the dish, swooning. Jesus Christ, before sitting down, let go in three regular and slamming sec. --The Gun party! ... That is to say that it starts! Then, gathering, he made a fourth, lonely, huge, offensive. --For Those nags of Buteau! they clog the mouth with! So Fouan dark since his arrival, sneered.

He approved a motion of the head. That put him at ease, they quoted it as a prankster, he as in his time; and in his home, the children had grown up, quiet in the middle of the paternal bombardment. He put his elbows on the table, he let himself invade wellness, opposite the great devil Jesus Christ, who gazed at him, his eyes moist, his air rabble good child. --Ah! name of God! Dad, we're going to take it easy! You see my thing, I undertake désemmerder you, me! ... When you Dining earth with moles, is it you advance, you be denied a fine piece? Shaken in the simplicity of his life, with the need to stun, Fouan finally said the same. --Well Sure it would be better to eat them that leaving nothing to other .... To your health, boy! Slutty veal served with onions.

There was a silence, and Jesus Christ, not to let the conversation drop in a shot extended, that crossed the straw from his chair with the modulation singing a human cry. Immediately, he turned to his daughter, serious and Interrogator: -- What Are you saying? She said nothing, she had to sit down, holding her stomach. But who finished it was after the calf and cheese last expansion father and son, who had started smoking and empty liter eau-de-vie, on the table. They no longer spoke, slurred mouth very drunk. Slowly, Jesus raised a buttock, thundered, then looked at the door, crying: --Come In!

So Fouan provoked angry at length not to be returned to its youth, high buttock, thundering in turn, replied: --Me Blowin! Both are slapped in the hands, face to face, drooling and laughing. It was good. And it was in too for Funk, who had slipped ground, stirred a frantic laugh to the point that in the shaking, she also let out a but light, thin and musical, as its Fife, next to the organ notes of the two men. Outraged, disgusted, Jesus Christ had risen, arm outstretched in a gesture tragic authority. --Hors Here, bitch! ... Get out of here, stink! ... Damn! I'll teach you to respect your father and your grandfather! He had never allowed him this familiarity. Had to have age. And hunting air by hand, affecting to be suffocated by this small flute breath: his, he said, did not feel that the powder. Then, as the culprit, very red, upset his forgetfulness, and denied fighting not to go out, he threw out a push. Large dirty --Bougre, shakes your skirts!... You do get back in a now, when you have taken the air.

But when the father and son got along, it was in their hatred of bailiff, Mr. Vimeux, a small shabby bailiff of being loaded chores with his colleague Cloyes would not, and ventured a evening testify at Chateau meaning of judgment. Vimeux was a man of unclean end, a yellow beard package, which only came out a red nose and bleary eyes. Always dressed in gentleman, a hat, a coat, a black pants, wear and abominable spots, he was famous in the township, for the terrible beatings he farmers received whenever he was forced to instrument against them, far from help.

Legends ran, saplings broken on his shoulders, baths forced to the bottom of ponds, a romp two kilometers with pitchforks, a spanking administered by the mother and daughter, panties down. Precisely, Jesus Christ returned with his gun; and Fouan father, smoking his pipe, sitting on a tree trunk, said in a growl angry: --Voilà Disgrace that you bring us, rascal! --Attendez See! murmured the poacher, through clenched teeth. But on seeing him with a gun, Vimeux had stopped short at a no thirties. All his pathetic person, black, dirty and correct, trembling with fear.

She said: Mr. Jesus Christ, he said a little thin voice, I come to the case, you know .... And I put it there. Good evening! It was filed on stamped paper on a stone, he went already backwards, strongly, while the other shouted: --The Name of God ink shit disturber, should we teach you manners! ... Will you give me your paper! And, like the poor, immobilized, frightened, did not dare either to advance or back an inch, he took aim. --I Send you lead, if you do not hurry up .... Come, return on your paper, and arrives .... Closer, closer, closer, but so damn capon, or I'll shoot!

Glossy, pale, Usher tottering on her short legs. He implored a look Fouan the father. It continued to quietly smoking his pipe, in his fierce grudge against the court costs and the man who embodies the eyes of the peasants. --Ah! here we are finally, it is not unhappy. Give me your paper. I Will Not! not the fingertips, as if reluctantly. Politely, dammit! and good heart .... There! you're nice. Vimeux, paralyzed by the sneers of this great guy, waiting in blinked under the threat of the joke, the punch or the slap, he felt it coming. --Now, Turn around.

He understood, did not move, clenched buttocks. --Retourne Up or I look back! He saw that he had to resign. Lamentable, he turned it presented himself behind her poor little lean cat. The other, Then, taking a spring, planted his foot in the right place, so steep, he sent it down on the nose, not four. And the bailiff, who fell painfully, galloped, distraught, hearing the cry --Watch Out! I'll shoot! Jesus Christ came to help. Only he merely raised the thigh, and bang! he snapped one, such a sound that terrified by detonation Vimeux fell flat again. This time, his black hat had rolled among the pebbles. He followed him, picked it up, ran harder. Behind him, the shots continued, bang! bang! bang! without a stop, a real shootout, amid loud laughter that make the finishing fool. Launched on the slope and an insect jumper, he was a hundred not already, that the echoes of the valley again repeated the cannonade Jesus Christ.

The entire campaign was full, and there was one last, great when the usher, shrunk to the size of an ant, there, disappeared in Rognes. Slutty, hastened to noise, holding his stomach, floor, giggling like a hen. The Fouan father had removed his pipe mouth to laugh more at ease. Ah! the name of God Jesus Christ! which not much! but fun all the same!

Famous Quotations:

"The stench of the manure that Jean was turning had cheered him up a little. He adored its promise of fertility and was sniffing it with the relish of a man smelling a randy woman."

"If you ask me what I came to do in this world, I, an artist, will answer you: I am here to live out loud."

"The artist is nothing without the gift, but the gift is nothing without work."

James Joyce

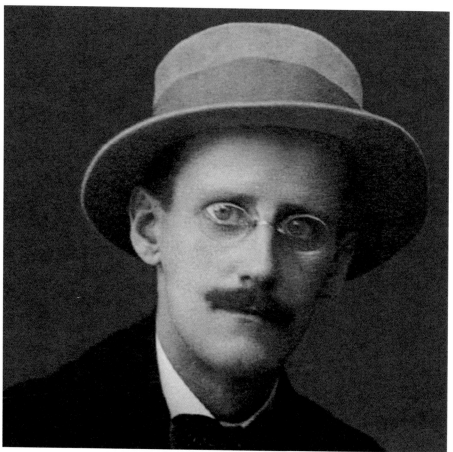

James Joyce, Public Domain

James Augustine Aloysius Joyce (1882 – 1941) was an Irish novelist and poet. In the opening sections of his classic work *Ulysses* there is the description of Leopold Bloom "as quat the cuckstool...seated calm above his own rising smell."
If you ever thought that your private correspondence might be seen in public you might be more circumspect about what you write. James Joyce, in a private letter addressed to "my sweet little whorish Nora, you had an arse full of farts that night, darling, and I fucked them out of you, big fat fellows, long windy ones, quick

little merry cracks and a lot of tiny little naughty farties ending in a long gush from your hole. It is wonderful to fuck a farting woman when every fuck drives one out of her. I think I would know Nora's fart anywhere.

I think I could pick hers out in a roomful of farting women. It is a rather girlish noise not like the wet windy fart which I imagine fat wives have. It is sudden and dry and dirty like what a bold girl would let off in fun in a school dormitory at night. I hope Nora will let off no end of her farts in my face so that I may know their smell also."

From his personal letter writing it is clear that James Joyce had a condition known as eproctophilia. Eproctophilia is a fart fetish, the receiving of sexual pleasure and arousal from the fart of another. As with many other authors, having a peculiar side interest did not diminish the quality of their professional writings.

Famous Quotations:

"Think you're escaping and run into yourself. Longest way round is the shortest way home."
"Shut your eyes and see."
"A man of genius makes no mistakes. His errors are volitional and are the portals of discovery."
"All Moanday, Tearday, Wailsday, Thumpsday, Frightday, Shatterday."
"Your battles inspired me - not the obvious material battles but those that were fought and won behind your forehead."
"I am tomorrow, or some future day, what I establish today. I am today what I established yesterday or some previous day."
"He wanted to cry quietly but not for himself: for the words, so beautiful and sad, like music."
"Secrets, silent, stony sit in the dark palaces of both our hearts: secrets weary of their tyranny: tyrants willing to be dethroned."
"One by one they were all becoming shades. Better pass boldly into that other world, in the full glory of some passion, than fade and wither dismally with age."
"My mouth is full of decayed teeth and my soul of decayed ambitions."
"Life is too short to read a bad book."
"Thus the unfacts, did we possess them, are too imprecisely few to warrant our certitude..."
"Have read little and understood less."
"There's no friends like the old friends."
"To learn one must be humble. But life is the great teacher."
"What's yours is mine and what's mine is my own."
"In the particular is contained the universal."
"Your mind will give back exactly what you put into it."
"There is not past, no future; everything flows in an eternal present."
"From the sublime to the ridiculous is but a step."

"Gazing up into the darkness I saw myself as a creature driven and derided by vanity; and my eyes burned with anguish and anger."

"History ... is a nightmare from which I am trying to wake."

"When a man is born...there are nets flung at it to hold it back from flight. You talk to me of nationality, language, religion. I shall try to fly by those nets."

"Pride and hope and desire like crushed herbs in his heart sent up vapours of maddening incense before the eyes of his mind."

"It is as painful perhaps to be awakened from a vision as to be born."

"Whatever else is unsure in this stinking dunghill of a world a mother's love is not."

"I care not if I live but a day and a night, so long as my deeds live after me."

"The demand that I make of my reader is that he should devote his whole life to reading my works."

"Don't eat a beefsteak. If you do the eyes of that cow will pursue you through all eternity."

"She said he just looked as if he was asleep, he looked that peaceful and resigned. No one would think he'd make such a beautiful corpse."

"While you have a thing it can be taken from you.....but when you give it, you have given it. no robber can take it from you. It is yours then forever when you have given it. It will be yours always. That is to give."

"I wanted real adventures to happen to myself. But real adventures, I reflected, do not happen to people who remain at home: they must be sought abroad."

"Read your own obituary notice; they say you live longer. Gives you second wind. New lease of life."

"Time is, time was, but time shall be no more."

"There is no heresy or no philosophy which is so abhorrent to the church as a human being."

"First we feel. Then we fall."

"Hold to the now, the here, through which all future plunges to the past."

D. H. Lawrence

David Herbert Lawrence (1885 –1930) was an English novelist, poet, playwright, essayist, literary critic and painter who published as D. H. Lawrence.

From *Sons and Lovers*, Chapter 3:
But they loved the Guild. It was the only thing to which they did not grudge their mother--and that partly because she enjoyed it, partly because of the treats they derived from it. The Guild was called by some hostile husbands, who found their wives getting too independent, the "clat-fart" shop--that is, the gossip-shop. It is true, from off the basis of the Guild, the women could look at their homes, at the conditions of their own lives, and find fault.

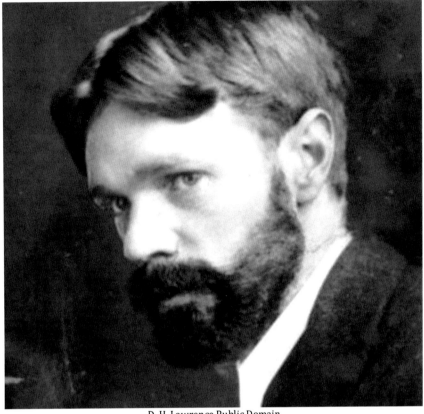
D. H. Lawrence Public Domain

Famous Quotations:

"A woman has to live her life, or live to repent not having lived it."
"All people dream, but not equally. Those who dream by night in the dusty recesses of their mind, wake in the morning to find that it was vanity. But the dreamers of the day are dangerous people, For they dream their dreams with open eyes, And make them come true."
"Life is ours to be spent, not to be saved."
"I want to live my life so that my nights are not full of regrets."
"I can never decide whether my dreams are the result of my thoughts or my thoughts the result of my dreams."
"Sleep is still most perfect, in spite of hygienists, when it is shared with a beloved."

Aldous Huxley

Aldous Huxley (1894-1963) was an English novelist, philosopher, humanist, pacifist, and satirist. His most famous work is the novel *Brave New World.*

In his work *Ape and Essence*:
"...reason comes running, eager to ratify, comes, a catch-fart with Philosophy, truckling to tyrants..."

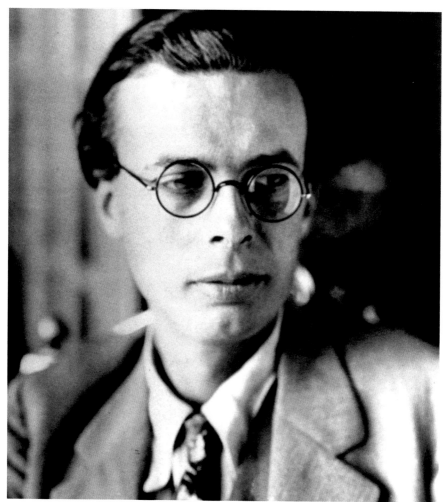
Aldous Huxley, Public Domain

Famous Quotations:

"For at least two thirds of our miseries spring from human stupidity, human malice and those great motivators and justifiers of malice and stupidity, idealism, dogmatism and proselytizing zeal on behalf of religious or political idols"
"We shall be permitted to live on this planet only for as long as we treat all nature with compassion and intelligence."
"Never put off till tomorrow the fun you can have today."

"Facts do not cease to exist because they are ignored."

"Habit converts luxurious enjoyments into dull and daily necessities."

"After silence, that which comes nearest to expressing the inexpressible is music."

"I want to know what passion is. I want to feel something strongly."

"The propagandist's purpose is to make one set of people forget that certain other sets of people are human."

"No social stability without individual stability."

"Most human beings have an almost infinite capacity for taking things for granted."

"Experience teaches only the teachable."

"Technological progress has merely provided us with more efficient means for going backwards."

"It's a little embarrassing that after 45 years of research & study, the best advice I can give people is to be a little kinder to each other."

"It isn't a matter of forgetting. What one has to learn is how to remember and yet be free of the past."

"We cannot reason ourselves out of our basic irrationality. All we can do is learn the art of being irrational in a reasonable way."

"The vast majority of human beings dislike and even actually dread all notions with which they are not familiar... Hence it comes about that at their first appearance innovators have generally been persecuted, and always derided as fools and madmen."

"I wanted to change the world. But I have found that the only thing one can be sure of changing is oneself."

"The Bhagavad-Gita is the most systematic statement of spiritual evolution of endowing value to mankind. It is one of the most clear and comprehensive summaries of perennial philosophy ever revealed; hence its enduring value is subject not only to India but to all of humanity."

"A child-like man is not a man whose development has been arrested; on the contrary, he is a man who has given himself a chance of continuing to develop long after most adults have muffled themselves in the cocoon of middle-aged habit and convention."

"An intellectual is a person who has discovered something more interesting than sex."

"That men do not learn very much from the lessons of history is the most important of all the lessons that history has to teach."

"Experience is not what happens to a man; it is what a man does with what happens to him."

"The secret of genius is to carry the spirit of the child into old age, which means never losing your enthusiasm."

"Chronic remorse, as all the moralists are agreed, is a most undesirable sentiment. If you have behaved badly, repent, make what amends you can and address yourself to the task of behaving better next time. On no account brood over your wrongdoing. Rolling in the muck is not the best way of getting clean."

"That all men are equal is a proposition which at ordinary times no sane individual has ever given his assent."

"All that happens means something; nothing you do is ever insignificant."

"The surest way to work up a crusade in favor of some good cause is to promise people they will have a chance of maltreating someone. To be able to destroy with good conscience, to be able to behave badly and call your bad behavior 'righteous indignation' — this is the height of psychological luxury, the most delicious of moral treats."

"Happiness is not achieved by the conscious pursuit of happiness; it is generally the by-product of other activities."

"There is only one corner of the universe you can be certain of improving, and that's your own self."

"One believes things because one has been conditioned to believe them."

"Ironically enough, the only people who can hold up indefinitely under the stress of modern war are psychotics. Individual insanity is immune to the consequences of collective insanity."

"Every man....who knows how to read, has it in his power to magnify himself, to multiply the ways in which he exists, to make his life full, significant and interesting."

"You never see animals going through the absurd and often horrible fooleries of magic and religion.... Dogs do not ritually urinate in the hope of persuading heaven to do the same and send down rain. Asses do not bray a liturgy to cloudless skies. Nor do cats attempt, by abstinence from cat's meat, to wheedle the feline spirits into benevolence. Only man behaves with such gratuitous folly. It is the price he has to pay for being intelligent but not, as yet, quite intelligent enough."

"One third, more or less, of all the sorrow that the person I think I am must endure is unavoidable. It is the sorrow inherent in the human condition, the price we must pay for being sentient and self-conscious organisms, aspirants to liberation, but subject to the laws of nature and under orders to keep on marching, through irreversible time, through a world wholly indifferent to our well-being, toward decrepitude and the certainty of death. The remaining two thirds of all sorrow is homemade and, so far as the universe is concerned, unnecessary."

"The real hopeless victims of mental illness are to be found among those who appear to be most normal. "Many of them are normal because they are so well adjusted to our mode of existence, because their human voice has been silenced so early in their lives, that they do not even struggle or suffer or develop symptoms as the neurotic does." They are normal not in what may be called the absolute sense of the word; they are normal only in relation to a profoundly abnormal society. Their perfect adjustment to that abnormal society is a measure of their mental sickness. These millions of abnormally normal people, living without fuss in a society to which, if they were fully human beings, they ought not to be adjusted."

Henry Miller

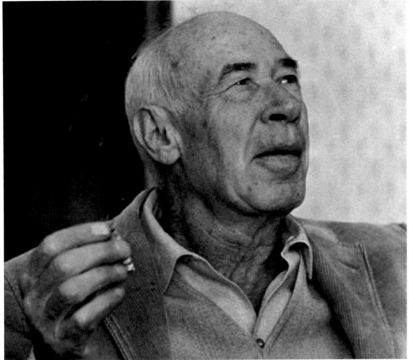

Henry Miller www.organicinsan.com

Henry Miller (1891 – 1980) was an American author, whose use of explicit language in his novels, especially *Tropic of Cancer*, led to court cases addressing the role of censorship in literature, including the banning of publication of written works.

In *Tropic of Cancer* he describes the positioning of a woman, as "she seemed to have slightly raised her ass from the sofa, as if to let a loud fart".

Famous Quotations:

"For the moment I can think of nothing— except that I am a sentient being stabbed by the miracle of these waters that reflect a forgotten world."
"The imperfections of a man, his frailties, his faults, are just as important as his virtues. You can't separate them. They're wedded."
"The one thing we can never get enough of is love. And the one thing we never give enough of is love."

"Conditioned to ecstasy, the poet is like a gorgeous unknown bird mired in the ashes of thought. If he succeeds in freeing himself, it is to make a sacrificial flight to the sun. His dreams of a regenerate world are but the reverberations of his own fevered pulse beats. He imagines the world will follow him, but in the blue he finds himself alone. Alone but surrounded by his creations; sustained, therefore, to meet the supreme sacrifice. The impossible has been achieved; the duologue of author with Author is consummated. And now forever through the ages the song expands, warming all hearts, penetrating all minds. At the periphery the world is dying away; at the center it glows like a live coal. In the great solar heart of the universe the golden birds are gathered in unison. There it is forever dawn, forever peace, harmony and communion. Man does not look to the sun in vain; he demands light and warmth not for the corpse which he will one day discard but for his inner being. His greatest desire is to burn with ecstasy, to commerge his little flame with the central fire of the universe. If he accords the angels wings so that they may come to him with messages of peace, harmony and radiance from worlds beyond, it is only to nourish his own dreams of flight, to sustain his own belief that he will one day reach beyond himself, and on wings of gold. One creation matches another; in essence they are all alike. The brotherhood of man consists not in thinking alike, nor in acting alike, but in aspiring to praise creation. The song of creation springs from the ruins of earthly endeavor. The outer man dies away in order to reveal the golden bird which is winging its way toward divinity."

Ernest Hemingway

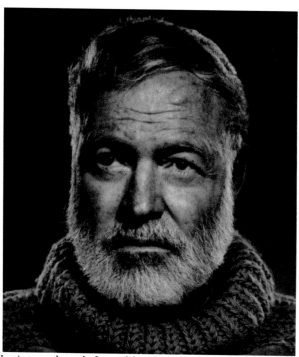

Ernest Hemingway throughaforestofideas.blogspot.com Creative Commons License

Ernest Hemingway (1899 – 1961 was an American author and journalist who was awarded the Nobel Prize in Literature in 1954. He lived a colorful and adventurous life that ended in suicide at the age of sixty one.

Many of his works are considered classics of American Literature. The following selection from *88 Poems* do not fall into the category of his classic writings.

"Home is where the heart is, home is where the fart is.
Come let us fart in the home.
There is no art in a fart.
Still a fart may not be artless.
Let us fart and artless fart in the home."

Famous Quotations:

"There is nothing noble in being superior to your fellow man; true nobility is being superior to your former self."
"There is no friend as loyal as a book."
"When people talk, listen completely. Most people never listen."
"It is good to have an end to journey toward; but it is the journey that matters, in the end."
"Courage is grace under pressure."
"Never confuse movement with action."
"you can't get away from yourself by moving from one place to another."
"Religion is the opium of the poor"
"When you stop doing things for fun you might as well be dead."
"Cowards die a thousand deaths, but the brave only die once."
"The most essential gift for a good writer is a built-in, shockproof, shit detector."
"If you are lucky enough to have lived in Paris as a young man, then wherever you go for the rest of your life, it stays with you, for Paris is a moveable feast."

Thomas Wolfe

Thomas Wolfe (1900-1938) was an American novelist who was known for his highly original impressionistic, and highly analytical prose. He is considered one if the most important writers in modern American literature. He was widely acclaimed during his lifetime and his influence was said to extend to many of the illustrious authors of his generation.

The phrase "a fizzing and sulphuric fart" was cut out of Thomas Wolfe's 1929 novel *Look Homeward, Angel* by his publisher because of censorship concerns. The novel; is considered to be highly autobiographical.

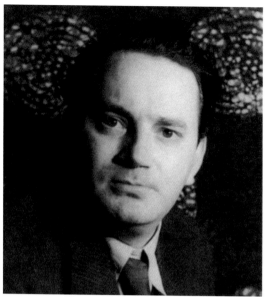
Thomas Wolfe, Public Domain

Famous Quotations:

"Man is born to live, to suffer, and to die, and what befalls him is a tragic lot. There is no denying this in the final end. But we must deny it all along the way."

"The whole conviction of my life now rests upon the belief that loneliness, far from being a rare and curious phenomenon, is the central and inevitable fact of human existence."

"I don't know yet what I am capable of doing, but, by God, I have genius -- I know it too well to blush behind it."

"Something has spoken to me in the night...and told me that I shall die, I know not where. Saying: "[Death is] to lose the earth you know for greater knowing; to lose the life you have, for greater life; to leave the friends you loved, for greater loving; to find a land more kind than home, more large than earth."

"We are the sum of all our parts"

"A sect, incidentally, is a religion with no political power."

"You have reached the pinnacle of success as soon as you become uninterested in money, compliments, or publicity."

"If a man has a talent and cannot use it, he has failed. If he has a talent and only uses half of it, he has partly failed. If he has a talent and learns to use the whole of it, he has gloriously succeeded, and won a satisfaction and triumph few men will know."

"This is man: a writer of books, a putter-down of words, a painter of pictures, a maker of ten thousand philosophies. He grows passionate over ideas, he hurls scorn and mockery at another's work, he finds the one way, the true way, for himself, and calls all others false--yet in the billion books upon the shelves there is not one that can tell him how to draw a single fleeting breath in peace and comfort. He makes histories of the universe, he directs the destiny of the nations, but he does not know his own history, and he cannot direct his own destiny with dignity or wisdom for ten consecutive minutes."

"Of all I have ever seen or learned, that book seems to me the noblest, the wisest, and the most powerful expression of man's life upon this earth — and also the highest flower of poetry, eloquence, and truth. I am not given to dogmatic judgments in the matter of literary creation, but if I had to make one I could say that Ecclesiastes is the greatest single piece of writing I have ever known, and the wisdom expressed in it the most lasting and profound."

"You can't go back home to your family, back home to your childhood, back home to romantic love, back home to a young man's dreams of glory and of fame, back home to exile, to escape to Europe and some foreign land, back home to lyricism, to singing just for singing's sake, back home to aestheticism, to one's youthful idea of 'the artist' and the all-sufficiency of 'art' and 'beauty' and 'love,' back home to the ivory tower, back home to places in the country, to the cottage in Bermude, away from all the strife and conflict of the world, back home to the father you have lost and have been looking for, back home to someone who can help you, save you, ease the burden for you, back home to the old forms and systems of things which once seemed everlasting but which are changing all the time--back home to the escapes of Time and Memory."

W.H. Auden

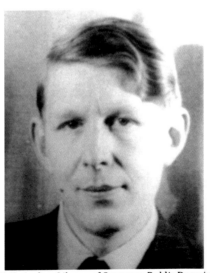

W. H. Auden, Library of Congress, Public Domain

Wystan Hugh Auden (1907 – 1973) was an Anglo American poet considered by many as one of the twentieth centuries greatest writers.

"Most people enjoy the sight of their own handwriting as they enjoy the smell of their own farts."

Famous Quotations:

"Poetry might be defined as the clear expression of mixed feelings."
"A poet is, before anything else, a person who is passionately in love with language."
"Among those whom I like or admire, I can find no common denominator, but among those whom I love, I can; all of them make me laugh."
"Whatever you do, good or bad, people will always have something negative to say"
"Poetry makes nothing happen."
"Language is the mother, not the handmaiden, of thought; words will tell you things you never thought or felt before."
"I used to try and concentrate the poem so much that there wasn't a word that wasn't essential. This leads to becoming boring and constipated."
"I used to try and concentrate the poem so much that there wasn't a word that wasn't essential. This leads to becoming boring and constipated."
"Aphorisms are essentially an aristocratic genre of writing. The aphorist does not argue or explain, he asserts; and implicit in his assertion is a conviction that he is wiser and more intelligent than his readers."
"The underlying reason for writing is to bridge the gulf between one person and another."

Roald Dahl

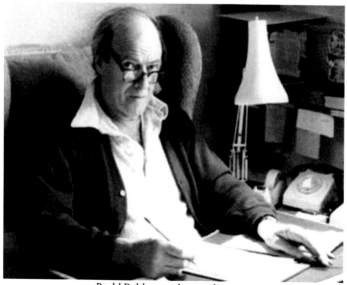

Roald Dahl www.thegaurdian.com

Roald Dahl (1916-1990) was an English novelist, poet, and fighter pilot who became one of the 20th century's favorite authors of children's books.

In *The BFG* the character The Big Friendly Giant engages in an activity described as whizzpopping, the passing of intestinal gas, at formal events. The giants believe burps are disgusting, and they love farting. They drink frobscottle, which makes the bubbles go down, instead of up. The following passages say it all:

"With frobscottle," Sophie said, "the bubbles in your tummy will be going downwards and that could have a far nastier result." "Why nasty?" asked the BFG, frowning. "Because," Sophie said, blushing a little, "if they go down instead of up, they'll be coming out somewhere else with an even louder and ruder noise."

"A whizzpopper!" cried the BFG, beaming at her. "Us giants is making whizzpoppers all the time! Whizzpopping is a sign of happiness. It is music in our ears! You surely is not telling me that a little whizzpopping is forbidden among human beans?"

"It is considered extremely rude," Sophie said. "But you is whizzpopping, is you not, now and again?" asked the BFG.

"Everyone is whizzpopping, if that's what you call it," Sophie said. "Kings and Queens are whizzpopping. Presidents are whizzpopping. Glamorous film stars are whizzpopping. Little babies are whizzpopping. But where I come from, it is not polite to talk about it."

"Redunculous!" said the BFG. "If everyone is making whizzpoppers, then why not talk about it? We is now having a swiggle of this delicious frobscottle and you will see the happy result."

The BFG shook the bottle vigorously. The pale green stuff fizzed and bubbled. He removed the cork and took a tremendous gurgling swig. "It's glummy!" he cried. "I love it!"

For a few moments, the Big Friendly Giant stood quite still, and a look of absolute ecstasy began to spread over his long wrinkly face. Then suddenly the heavens opened and he let fly with a series of the loudest and rudest noises Sophie had ever heard in her life.

They reverberated around the walls of the cave like thunder and the glass jars rattled on their shelves. But most astonishing of all, the force of the explosions actually lifted the enormous giant clear off his feet, like a rocket.

"Whoopee!" he cried, when he came down to earth again. "Now that is whizzpopping for you!"

Famous Quotations:

"You can write about anything for children as long as you've got humour."
"Never do anything by halves if you want to get away with it. Be outrageous..."

Samuel Beckett

Samuel Beckett (1906-1989) was Irish novelist, poet, theater director and playwright.

"[A]ll I want to do is sit on my ass and fart and think of Dante."

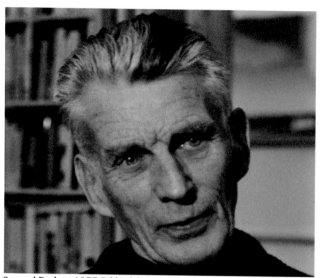

Samuel Beckett 1977 Bibliothèque nationale de France Public Domain

In Beckett's *Molloy'* there is a soliloquy about prodigious farting:
"Chameleon in spite of himself, there you have Molloy, viewed from a certain angle. And in winter, under my greatcoat, I wrapped myself in swathes of newspaper, and did not shed them until earth awoke, for good, in April. The Times Literary Supplement was admirably adapted to this purpose, of a never-failing toughness and impermeability. Even farts made no impression on it. I can't help it, gas escapes from my fundament on the least pretext, it's hard not to mention it now and then, however great my distaste.

One day I counted them. Three hundred and fifteen farts in nineteen hours, or an average of over sixteen farts an hour. After all it's not excessive. Four farts every fifteen minutes. It's nothing. Not even one fart every four minutes. It's unbelievable. Damn it, I hardly fart at all, I should never have mentioned it. Extraordinary how mathematics help you know yourself."

Famous Quotations:

"We are all born mad. Some remain so."
"All of old. Nothing else ever. Ever tried. Ever failed. No matter. Try again. Fail again. Fail better."
"Words are all we have."
"The creation of the world did not take place once and for all time, but takes place every day."
"Poets are the sense, philosophers the intelligence of humanity."
"Poets are the sense, philosophers the intelligence of humanity."
"We have time to grow old. The air is full of our cries. But habit is a great deadener."
"There is this to be said for Dachshunds of such length and lowness as Nelly, that it makes very little difference to their appearance whether they stand, sit or lie."
"Not one person in a hundred knows how to be silent and listen, no, nor even to conceive what such a thing means. Yet only then can you detect, beyond the fatuous clamor, the silence of which the universe is made."

J.D. Salinger

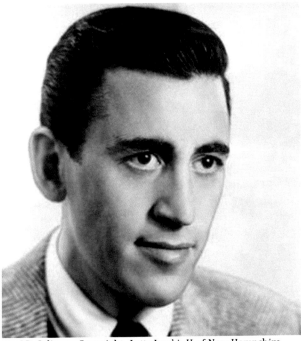

J.D. Salinger, Copyright, Lotte Jacobi, U. of New Hampshire.

Jerome David Salinger (1919 – 2010) was a reclusive American author whose work *Catcher in the Rye* is considered an American classic. Listening contemptuously to minister Ossenburger's self-aggrandizing sermon, Holden

Caulfield's scorn is temporarily interrupted when:

The Catcher in the Rye:
"This guy sitting in the row in front of me, Edgar Marsalla, laid this terrific fart. It was a very crude thing to do, in the chapel and all, but it was also quite amusing. Old Marsalla. He damn near blew the roof off."

Famous Quotations:

"The mark of the immature man is that he wants to die nobly for a cause, while the mark of the mature man is that he wants to live humbly for one."
"I'm a kind of paranoiac in reverse. I suspect people of plotting to make me happy."
"Know your true measurements and dress your mind accordingly"
"I'm quite illiterate, but I read a lot."
"Among other things, you'll find that you're not the first one who was ever confused and frightened and even sickened by human behavior."
"One day a long time from now you'll cease to care anymore whom you please or what anybody has to say about you. That's when you'll finally produce the work you're capable of."

Kurt Vonnegut, Jr.

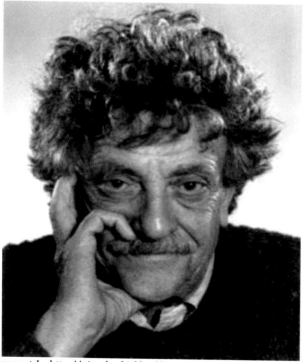

Kurt Vonnegut, Jr. http://ninasbookieblog.blogspot.com Creative Commons License

Kurt Vonnegut, Jr. (1922-2007) was an American author and humanist philosopher, who was known for his satire of the society in which he lived. His works included *Cat's Cradle*, *Slaughterhouse-Five*, and *Breakfast of Champions*. The *New York Times* labeled him as the counterculture's novelist

"I tell you, we are here on Earth to fart around, and don't let anybody tell you different." - Kurt Vonnegut

Famous Quotations:

"We have to continually be jumping off cliffs and developing our wings on the way down."
"Of all the words of mice and men, the saddest are, "It might have been.""
"Being a Humanist means trying to behave decently without expectation of rewards or punishment after you are dead."
"A sane person to an insane society must appear insane."
"Science is magic that works."
"If you can do no good, at least do no harm."
"All of the true things I am about to tell you are shameless lies."
"Beware of the man who works hard to learn something, learns it, and finds himself no wiser than before. He is full of murderous resentment of people who are ignorant without having come by their ignorance the hard way."
"A saint is a person who behaves decently in a shockingly indecent society."
"And a step backward, after making a wrong turn, is a step in the right direction."
"People say there are no atheists in foxholes. A lot of people think this is a good argument against atheism. Personally, I think it's a much better argument against foxholes."
"New knowledge is the most valuable commodity on earth. The more truth we have to work with, the richer we become."
"I believe that reading and writing are the most nourishing forms of meditation anyone has so far found. By reading the writings of the most interesting minds in history, we meditate with our own minds and theirs as well. This to me is a miracle."

Norman Mailer

Norman Mailer (1923 – 2007) was a Pulitzer Prize winning American author, journalist, and essayist whose work included the novel *The Naked and the Dead* and *The Executioner's Song*.

He wrote an essay entitled *We Know Everything About the Great But How They Fart.*

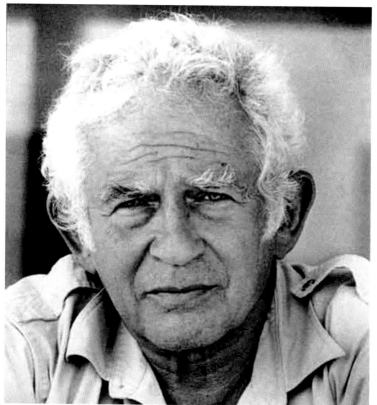

Norman Mailer www.peerie.com Creative Commons License

Famous Quotations:

"Writing books is the closest men ever come to childbearing."
"Ultimately a hero is a man who would argue with the gods, and so awakens devils to contest his vision. The more a man can achieve, the more he may be certain that the devil will inhabit a part of his creation."
"You don't know a woman until you've met her in court."
"The function of socialism is to raise suffering to a higher level."

The Gospel According to the Son:
"I am not here only so that the blind might see, but to teach those who thought they could see that they are blind"

William Styron

William Styron (1925- 2006) is an American author who won the Pulitzer Prize in Literature in 1967 for his novel *The Confessions of Nat Turner*. In the novel his attorney is interviewing the imprisoned black revolutionary.

The Confessions of Nat Turner:
"I saw Gray stir uncomfortably, then raise one haunch up off a fart trying to slide it out gracefully, but it emerged in multiple soft reports like the popping of remote firecrackers."

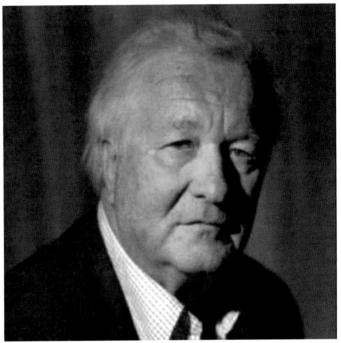

William Styron ww.nhtributes.com Creative Commons License

Famous Quotations:

"A great book should leave you with many experiences, and slightly exhausted at the end. You live several lives while reading."

"The pain of severe depression is quite unimaginable to those who have not suffered it, and it kills in many instances because its anguish can no longer be borne."

Sophie's Choice:
"*Someday I will understand Auschwitz.* This was a brave statement but innocently absurd. No one will ever understand Auschwitz. What I might have set down with more accuracy would have been: *Someday I will write about Sophie's life and death, and thereby help demonstrate how absolute evil is never extinguished from the world.* Auschwitz itself remains inexplicable. The most profound statement yet made about Auschwitz was not a statement at all, but a response.

The query: "At Auschwitz, tell me, where was God?"
And the answer: "Where was man?"

George MacDonald Fraser

George MacDonald Fraser (1925-2008) was a Scottish author who wrote historical novels, screenplays, and non-fiction books. He was honored by being made an Officer of the Order of the British Empire (OBE) in 1999.

He is most well known for his twelve volume series that featured the heroic character Flashman. Flashman's farting is legendary, most notably perhaps as he joined the Charge of the Light Brigade. He even managed to acquire the Apache name 'Wind-breaker' – the short form of his full name 'White-Rider-Goes-So-Fast-He-Destroys-the-Wind-with-His-Speed"...

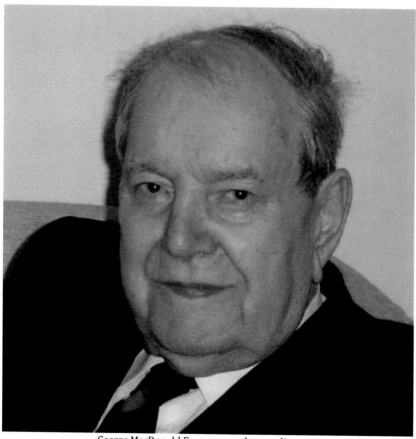
George MacDonald Fraser www.theguardian.com

Flashman at the Charge
"...and suddenly, without the slightest volition on my part, there was the most crashing discharge of wind, like the report of a mortar. My horse started; Cardigan jumped in his saddle, glaring at me.....Be Silent! snaps he, and he must have been

in a highly nervous condition himself, otherwise he would never have added, in a hoarse whisper: Can you not contain yourself, you disgusting fellow?--Flashman at the start of the Charge of the Light Brigade."

Famous Quotations:

"There's a point, you know, where treachery is so complete and unashamed that it becomes statesmanship."

"I've never been fool enough to confuse religion with belief in God. That's where so many clergymen...go wrong"

"If anything in their history demonstrates that the Scots are remarkable, it is that in spite of being physically attached to England, they have survived as a people, with their own culture, laws, institutions, and, like the English, their own ideas."

"England was a menace to Scotland because Scotland was, by its separate existence, a constant anxiety to England."

John Barth

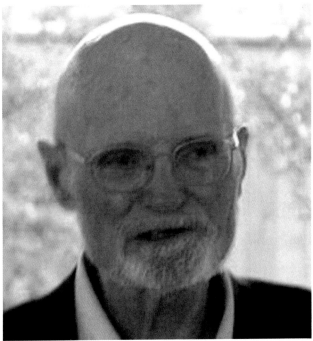

John Barth apocalypsebook.net

John Barth (1930 -) is an American author and professor known for his novels and short stories. In his 1960 post-modernist work *The Sot-Weed Factor* he provides a parody of the historical novel. The following passage provides an example of his writing in the style and various spellings of the 17th century.

"But this was a hard matter, inasmuch as for everrie cheerie wave of the hand I signaled them, some souldier of Gentleman in my companie must needs let goe a fart, which the Salvages did take as an affront, and threwe more arrows."

"Everyone is necessarily the hero of his own life story."

"The enemy you flee is not exterior to yourself"

"When you look at this mirror I hope you'll remember that there's always another way of seeing things: that's the beginning of wisdom."

"My feeling about technique in art is that it has about the same value as technique in lovemaking. That is to say, heartfelt ineptitude has its appeal and so does heartless skill; but what you want is passionate virtuosity."

"All men are loyal, but their objects of allegiance are at best approximate."

"I admire writers who can make complicated things simple, but my own talent has been to make simple things complicated."

John Kennedy Toole

John Kennedy Toole (1937- 1969) author of the Pulitzer Prize winning (1990) humorous novel *A Confederacy of Dunces*. The hero, Ignatius J Rielly, is an introverted intellectual who lives with his mother and is challenged in his dealings with contemporary society. To add to his emotional torment he is morbidly obese and burdened with a highly sensitive digestive tract that makes its presence known with intense bouts of flatulence. He blames his excessive farting on his mother's erratic driving and the absence of 'proper geometry and theology ' in the modern world.

A Confederacy of Dunces:
"It smells terrible in here.'

Well, what do you expect? The human body, when confined, produces certain odors which we tend to forget in this age of deodorants and other perversions. Actually, I find the atmosphere of this room rather comforting. Schiller needed the scent of apples rotting in his desk in order to write. I, too, have my needs. You may remember that Mark Twain preferred to lie supinely in bed while composing those rather dated and boring efforts which contemporary scholars try to prove meaningful. Veneration of Mark Twain is one of the roots of our current intellectual stalemate."

"The Dr. Nuts seemed only as an acid gurgling down into his intestine. He filled with gas, the sealed valve trapping it just as one pinches the mouth of a balloon. Great eructations rose from his throat and bounced upward toward the refuse-laden bowl of the milk glass chandelier."

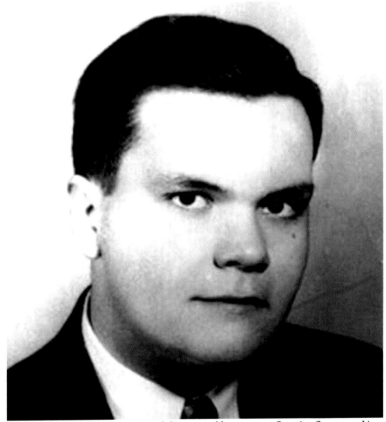

John Kennedy Toole www.mipatriaeslaliteratura.blogspot.com Creative Commons License

Famous Quotations:

"You can always tell employees of the government by the total vacancy which occupies the space where most other people have faces."
"Once a person was asked to step into this brutal century, anything could happen"
"Jail was preferable. There they only limited you physically. In a mental ward they tampered with your soul and worldview and mind."
"Dictatorship naturally arises out of democracy, and the most aggravated form of tyranny and slavery out of the most extreme liberty."

Philip Roth

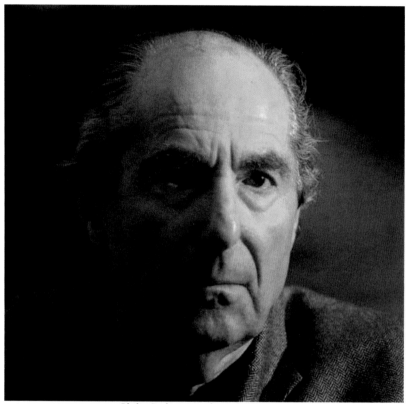

Philip Roth apieceofmonolopgue.com

Philip Roth (1933 -) is a Pulitzer Prize winning contemporary American author.

Portnoy's Complaint:
"When I fart in the bathtub, she kneels naked on the tile floor, leans all the way over, and kisses the bubbles."

The Great American Novel:
Kids love farts, don't they? Even today, with all the drugs and sex and violence you hear about on TV, they still get a kick, such as we used to, out of a fart. Maybe the world hasn't changed so much after all. It would be nice to think there were still a few eternal verities around. I hate to think of the day, when you say to an American kid, "Hey, want to smell a great fart?" and he looks at you as though you're crazy. "A great what ?" ""Fart. Don't you even know what a fart is? ""Sure it's a game—you throw one at a target. You get points." "That's a dart, dope. A fart. A bunch of kids sit around in a crowded place and they fart. Break wind. Sure, you can make it into a game and give points. So much for a wet fart, so much for a series, and so on. And penal-ties if you draw mud, as we called it in those days.

But the great thing was, you could do it just for the fun of it. By God, we could fart for hours when we were boys! Somebody's front porch on a warm summer night, in the road, on our way to school. Why, we could sit around a blacksmith's shop on a rainy day doing nothing but farting, and be perfectly content. No movies in those days. No television. No nothin'. I don't believe the whole bunch of us taken together ever had more than a nickel at any time, and yet we were never bored, never had to go around looking for excitement or getting into trouble. Best thing was you could do it yourself too. Yessir, boy knew how to make use of his leisure time in those days."

Surprising, given the impact of the fart on the life of the American boy, how little you still hear about it; from all appearances it is still something they'd rather skip over in The Canterbury Tales at Valhalla High. On the other hand, that may be a blessing in disguise; this way' at least no moneyman or politician has gotten it into his head yet to cash in on its nostalgic appeal. Because when that happens, you can kiss the fart good-bye. They will cheapen and degrade it until it is on a level with Mom's apple pie and our flag. Mark my words: as soon as some scoundrel discovers there is a profit to be made off of the American kid's love of the fart, they will be selling artificial farts in balloons at the circus. And you can just imagine what they'll smell like too. Like everything artificial.

Yes, fans, as the proverb has it, verily there is nothing like a case of fecal impaction to make an old man wax poetic about the fart. Forgive the sentimental meandering.

Famous Quotations:

"You put too much stock in human intelligence, it doesn't annihilate human nature."

"You cannot observe people through an ideology. Your ideology observes for you."

"I came to New York and in only hours, New York did what it does to people: awakened the possibilities. Hope breaks out."

"All that we don't know is astonishing. Even more astonishing is what passes for knowing."

"--nor had I understood til then how the shameless vanity of utter fools can so strongly determine the fate of others"

"Everyone becomes a part of history whether they like it or not and whether they know it or not."

"You can no more make someone tell the truth than you can force someone to love you."

"There is truth and then again there is truth. For all that the world is full of people who go around believing they've got you or your neighbor figured out, there really is no bottom to what is not known. The truth about us is endless. As are the lies."

"I'm interested in what people do with the chaos in their lives and how they respond to it, and simultaneously what they do with what they feel like are limitations. If they push against these limitations, will they wind up in the realm of chaos, or will they push against limitations and wind up in the world of freedom?"

"You have a conscience, and a conscience is a valuable attribute, but not if it begins to make you think you were to blame for what is far beyond the scope of your responsibility."

"It's human to have a secret, but it's just as human to reveal it sooner or later."

"He had learned the worst lesson that life can teach-that it makes no sense. And when that happens the happiness is never spontaneous again."

George Carlin

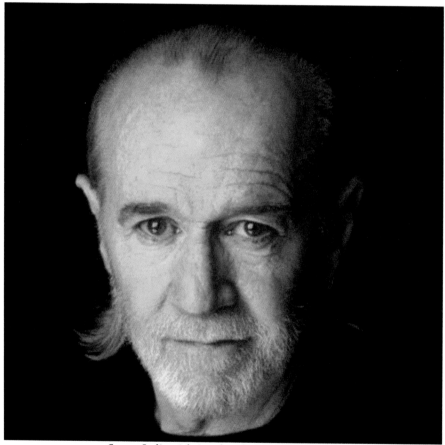

George Carlin mizbviewsfromthetower.blogspot.com

George Carlin (1937-2008) was an author, comedian and social critic. His satire and comedy routine on the 'seven dirty words' that were restricted from use on the public airways in the U.S. were subject to a Supreme Court decision affirming the governments right to regulate what the court considered indecent.

His material often included commentary about farts, mentioned in several of his books, including *Brain Droppings*. The except below is from one of his many stage performances:

Did you ever have to fart in a bus or on an airplane or in some other public place, but you hadn't been farting all that day. So you didn't really know the nature of the beast, you only knew there was lots of it. In a situation like that, what you have to do is release a test fart. You have to arrange to release quietly, and in a carefully controlled manner, about 10 to 15% of the total fart, in order to determine that those around you can handle it, or if you're about to precipitate a public health emergency. When releasing a test fart it is often good to engage in an act of subterfuge, such as reaching for a magazine. Say is that golf digest magazine, pfffffft.

That doesn't smell too horrifying, in fact in an odd way it's rather pleasant. I think they ought to enjoy the rest of this baby. And it turns out to be one of those farts that would skip the varnish off a footlocker, a fart that could end a marriage. And everyone around you heads to the exits, even the people on an airplane. As you realize it is time to review your fiber intake. It might not be necessary, after all, each morning to eat an entire wicker swing set.

Famous Quotations:

"The reason I talk to myself is because I'm the only one whose answers I accept."
"Those who dance are considered insane by those who cannot hear the music."
"Here's all you have to know about men and women: women are crazy, men are stupid. And the main reason women are crazy is that men are stupid."
"Think of how stupid the average person is, and realize half of them are stupider than that."
"I'm completely in favor of the separation of Church and State.... These two institutions screw us up enough on their own, so both of them together is certain death."
"Have you ever noticed that anybody driving slower than you is an idiot, and anyone going faster than you is a maniac?"
"Fighting for peace is like screwing for virginity."
"If you try to fail, and succeed, which have you done?"
"Never underestimate the power of stupid people in large groups."
"Some people see things that are and ask, Why?
Some people dream of things that never were and ask, Why not?
Some people have to go to work and don't have time for all that."
"Religion is like a pair of shoes.....Find one that fits for you, but don't make me wear your shoes."
"Don't just teach your children to read...
Teach them to question what they read.
Teach them to question everything."

"Never argue with an idiot. They will only bring you down to their level and beat you with experience."

"Inside every cynical person, there is a disappointed idealist."

"If lawyers are disbarred and clergymen defrocked, doesn't it follow that electricians can be delighted, musicians denoted?"

"Life is not measured by the breathes you take, but by the moments that take your breathe away."

"When it comes to God's existence, I'm not an atheist and I'm not agnostic. I'm an acrostic. The whole thing puzzles me."

"Trying to be happy by accumulating possessions is like trying to satisfy hunger by taping sandwiches all over your body."

"Always do whatever's next."

"Everyone smiles in the same language."

"Scratch any cynic and you will find a disappointed idealist."

"I went to a bookstore and asked the saleswoman, 'Where's the self-help section?' She said if she told me, it would defeat the purpose."

"Atheism is a non-prophet organization."

"Tell people there is an invisible man in the sky who created the universe, and the vast majority will believe you. Tell them the paint is wet, and they have to touch it to be sure."

"Honesty may be the best policy, but it's important to remember that apparently, by elimination, dishonesty is the second-best policy."

"In America, anyone can become president. That's the problem."

"Isn't making a smoking section in a restaurant, like making a peeing section in a swimming pool?"

"I think I am, therefore, I am... I think."

"The most unfair thing about life is the way it ends. I mean, life is tough. It takes up a lot of your time. What do you get at the end of it? A Death! What's that, a bonus? I think the life cycle is all backwards. You should die first, get it out of the way. Then you live in an old age home. You get kicked out when you're too young, you get a gold watch, you go to work. You work forty years until you're young enough to enjoy your retirement. You do drugs, alcohol, you party, you get ready for high school. You go to grade school, you become a kid, you play, you have no responsibilities, you become a little baby, you go back into the womb, you spend your last nine months floating ...and you finish off as an orgasm."

"Religion has actually convinced people that there's an invisible man living in the sky who watches everything you do, every minute of every day. And the invisible man has a special list of ten things he does not want you to do. And if you do any of these ten things, he has a special place, full of fire and smoke and burning and torture and anguish, where he will send you to live and suffer and burn and choke and scream and cry forever and ever 'til the end of time! But He loves you. He loves you, and He needs money! He always needs money! He's all-powerful, all-perfect, all-knowing, and all-wise, somehow just can't handle money!"

"I don't like ass kissers, flag wavers or team players. I like people who buck the system. Individualists. I often warn people: "Somewhere along the way, someone is going to tell you, 'There is no "I" in team.' What you should tell them is, 'Maybe not. But there is an "I" in independence, individuality and integrity.'" Avoid teams at all cost. Keep your circle small. Never join a group that has a name. If they say, "We're the So-and-Sos," take a walk. And if, somehow, you must join, if it's unavoidable, such as a union or a trade association, go ahead and join. But don't participate; it will be your death. And if they tell you you're not a team player, congratulate them on being observant."

Sir Salman Rushdie

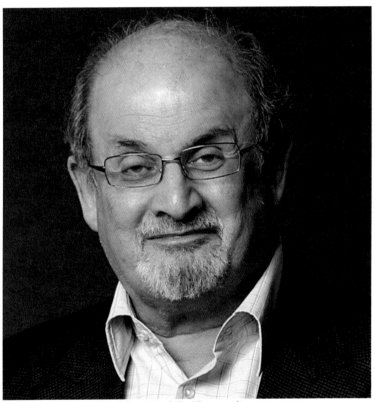

Sir Salman Rushdie The guardian.com

Sir Salman Rushdie (1947-) is an acclaimed award winning British Indian novelist and essayist of Muslim descent. His work is described as a combination of magical realism and historical fiction. His volume *The Satanic Verses* provoked protests from a number of Muslims, including the Ayatollah Ruhollah Khomeini, the Supreme Leader of Iran. Khomeini did not read the book, nonetheless as the leader of an Islamic theocracy issued a decree known as a *fatwā* calling for Rushdie's assassination.

Objections to the literal death sentence were condemned by Western society, but the decree remains an active assassination order with many religious adherents vowing to fulfill it at the first opportunity. After the death of Ayatollah Khomeini the Ayatollah who became the next Supreme Leader of Iran reaffirmed the *fatwā*, and again called for Rushdie's assassination. He has since written a book *Joseph Antoin: A Memoir* describing his experience as the target of assassination in an attempt at censorship from religious authorities abroad.

Shalimar the Clown
"... learning the knack of disconnecting her sense of smell, until she could switch it off like a radio and in the bland silence of its absence could drown in the sound of Nazarébaddoor's hypnotic voice without having her reverie interrupted by the scent of sheep shit or Nazarébaddoor's own frequent and extraordinary buffalo farts."

Famous Quotations:

"Language is courage: the ability to conceive a thought, to speak it, and by doing so to make it true."
"Faith without doubt is addiction"
"The moment you say that any idea system is sacred, whether it's a religious belief system or a secular ideology, the moment you declare a set of ideas to be immune from criticism, satire, derision, or contempt, freedom of thought becomes impossible."
"The inevitable triumph of illusion over reality that was the single most obvious truth about the history of the human race."
"The lessons one learns at school are not always the ones the school thinks it's teaching."
"Life is lived forward but is judged in reverse."
"Fundamentalism isn't about religion, it's about power."
"Vertigo is the conflict between the fear of falling and the desire to fall."
"Free societies..are societies in motion, and with motion comes tension, dissent, friction. Free people strike sparks, and those sparks are the best evidence of freedom's existence."
"Now I know what a ghost is. Unfinished business, that's what."
"What is freedom of expression? Without the freedom to offend, it ceases to exist."
"You can't judge an internal injury by the size of the hole."
"What can't be cured must be endured."
"We all owe death a life."
"Most of what matters in our lives takes place in our absence."
"The only people who see the whole picture,' he murmured, 'are the ones who step out of the frame."
"A poet's work . . . to name the unnamable, to point at frauds, to take sides, start arguments, shape the world and stop it from going to sleep."

"From the beginning men used God to justify the unjustifiable."
"What's real and what's true aren't necessarily the same."

"Our lives disconnect and reconnect, we move on, and later we may again touch one another, again bounce away. This is the felt shape of a human life, neither simply linear nor wholly disjunctive nor endlessly bifurcating, but rather this bouncey-castle sequence of bumpings-into and tumblings-apart."

"Memory has its own special kind. It selects, eliminates, alters, exaggerates, minimizes, glorifies, and vilifies also; but in the end it creates its own reality, its heterogeneous but usually coherent version of events; and no sane human being ever trusts someone else's version more than his own."

"I am the sum total of everything that went before me, of all I have been seen done, of everything done-to-me. I am everyone everything whose being-in-the-world affected was affected by mine. I am anything that happens after I'm gone which would not have happened if I had not come."

"What kind of idea are you? Are you the kind that compromises, does deals, accommodates itself to society, aims to find a niche, to survive; or are you the cussed, bloody-minded, ramrod-backed type of damnfool notion that would rather break than sway with the breeze? – The kind that will almost certainly, ninety-nine times out of hundred, be smashed to bits; but, the hundredth time, will change the world."

"Go for broke. Always try and do too much. Dispense with safety nets. Take a deep breath before you begin talking. Aim for the stars. Keep grinning. Be bloody-minded. Argue with the world. And never forget that writing is as close as we get to keeping a hold on the thousand and one things--childhood, certainties, cities, doubts, dreams, instants, phrases, parents, loves--that go on slipping, like sand, through our fingers."

"Nobody has the right to not be offended. That right doesn't exist in any declaration I have ever read. If you are offended it is your problem, and frankly lots of things offend lots of people. I can walk into a bookshop and point out a number of books that I find very unattractive in what they say. But it doesn't occur to me to burn the bookshop down. If you don't like a book, read another book. If you start reading a book and you decide you don't like it, nobody is telling you to finish it. To read a 600-page novel and then say that it has deeply offended you: well, you have done a lot of work to be offended."

James Patterson

James Patterson (1947 -) is an American author who has written novels that have sold over 300 million copies. One of his most popular fictional characters is the psychologist Alex Cross.

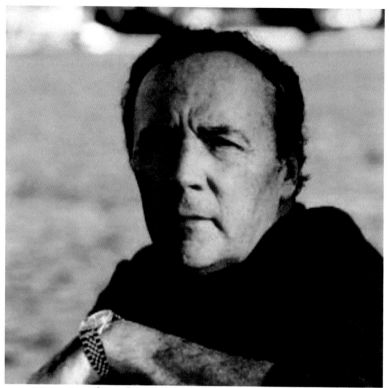

James Patterson www.librarything.com/pic

Max:
"We try not to encourage demonstrations of his mastery of the gaseous arts."

Fang:
Fang telling me stupid fart jokes from the dog crate next to mine at the school, trying to make me laugh.

The Final Warning:
"I want to do it too!" said Gazzy, sitting very, very quietly, completely motionless.
"Nope," said Nudge, shaking her head. "You stand out like a fart in church."
"Uh-oh,' said Gazzy, but Angel was so nauseated she didn't have time to leap to a safe distance, or grab a gas mask. Bbbbbrrrrrrrrttthhhhhhhttttttt.
'Mother of God, no!' Total cried, doing a fast belly-crawl to the pool and throwing himself in. 'You said it wasn't your digestive system!'
'What was that?' Dylan asked. He winced and threw an arm oer his nose and mouth. Sorry,' Gazzy said miserably, but he couldn't help a tiny grin.
Nudge was clawing at a stack of towels to cover her face. 'Nice one, Gaz,' said Iggy.
'Wait-that was Gazzy? Is that why you call him...Oh, crap,' Dylan said weakly."

Famous Quotations:

"If your going to look back on something and laugh about it, you might as well laugh about it now."
"The funny thing about facing imminent death is that it really snaps everything else into perspective."
"Honesty is always good, except when it's better to lie. "
"What are we but our stories?"
"Knowledge is a terrible burden. It may help you, but it might also destroy you."
"People always remember the worst day of their lifes. It becomes a part of them forever."
"You are an endless project...changing, evolving, surprising."
"Life is a great big canvas. Throw all the paint you can at it."
"Never underestimate the power of funny, it moves mountains."
"There's nothing more dangerous than someone trying to act for the greater good."
"The weird, weird thing about devastating loss is that life actually goes on."
"Denial is not just a river in Egypt."
"We is always so much better than I."
"The trick to having obedient, unquestioning children was to have death be the other option"
"Don't depend on others to give you strength....Find it within yourself"
"Everything I loved was taken away from me, and I did not die."
"you plan to fail if you fail to plan"
"I watched the way our fingers intertwined, and I thought, What are hands made for but this? For holding. For holding on."
"There are some feelings, and actions, for which words are utterly useless."
"I had made a friend. My second one in fourteen years. I was on a roll"
"Speed never killed anyone! It's suddenly becoming stationary... that's what gets you."
"Failure isn't falling down, it's staying down."
"You must do today what nobody else will do, so tomorrow you can accomplish what others can't."
"Nowhere will you meet more interesting people than in books."
"If you're going to look back on something and laugh about it, you might as well laugh about it now. Things are almost never as bad as they first seem."
"There's no such thing as a kid who hates reading. There are kids who love reading, and kids who are reading the wrong books."
"On the other hand, sometimes a happy delusion is better than grim reality."

Iain Banks

Iain Banks (1954-2013) was a Scottish author of the novel *The Wasp Factory*. In the novel the father can tell by his son's farts how much his alcoholic son has been drinking.

"'Well, just you be careful, then. I always know how much you've had from your farts.' He snorted, as though imitating one.

"My father has a theory about the link between mind and bowel being both crucial and very direct…. He has variously claimed that from farts he can tell not only what people have eaten or drunk, but also the sort of person they are, what they *ought* to eat, whether they are emotionally unstable or upset, whether they are keeping secrets, laughing at you behind your back or trying to ingratiate themselves with you, and even what they are thinking at the precise moment they issue the fart (this largely from the sound.) All total nonsense.

"'H'm,' I said, non-committal to a fault.

'Oh, I can,' he said as I finished my meal and leaned back, wiping my mouth on the back of my hand, more to annoy him than anything else. He kept nodding. 'I know when you've had Heavy or Lager. And I've smelt Guinness off you, too.'

"'I don't drink Guinness,' I lied, secretly impressed.'"

And later in the novel:

"'Brap!' said my anus loudly, surprising me as well as my father…I could see his nostrils flex and quiver.

"'Lager and whiskey, eh?'"

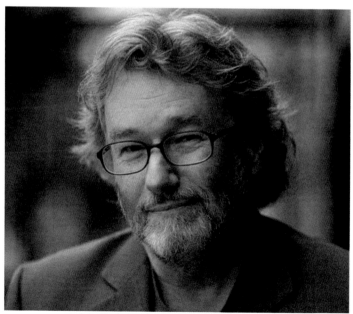

Iain Banks (1954-2013) www.thesun.co.uk

Famous Quotations:

"There are no gods, we are told, so I must make my own salvation."
"Empathize with stupidity and you're halfway to thinking like an idiot"
"The trouble with writing fiction is that it has to make sense, whereas real life doesn't."
"It's a library, only the stupid or the evil are afraid of those"
"I just think people overvalue argument because they like to hear themselves talk."
"Perdition awaits at the end of a road constructed entirely from good intentions, the devil emerges from the details and hell abides in the small print."
"My gratitude extends beyond the limits of my capacity to express it."
"Experience as well as common sense indicated that the most reliable method of avoiding self-extinction was not to equip oneself with the means to accomplish it in the first place."
"Reason shapes the future, but superstition infects the present."
"I think the easiest people to fool are ourselves. Fooling ourselves may even be a necessary precondition for fooling others."

"People can be teachers and idiots; they can be philosophers and idiots; they can be politicians and idiots... in fact I think they have to be... a genius can be an idiot. The world is largely run for and by idiots; it is no great handicap in life and in certain areas is actually a distinct advantage and even a prerequisite for advancement."

"There has seldom if ever a shortage of eager young males prepared to kill and die to preserve the security, comfort and prejudices of their elders, and what you call heroism is just an expression of this simple fact; there is never a scarcity of idiots."

"The truth is not always useful, not always good. It's like putting your faith in water. Yes, we need the rain, but too much can sweep you away in a flood and drown you. Like all great natural, elemental forces, the truth needs to be channeled, managed, controlled and intelligently, morally allocated."

Howard Stern

Howard Allan Stern (1954-) is an American author, actor, radio and television personality. His characteristic usage of material that may offend segments of the listening population has made him the most fined broadcaster in the history of the United States Federal Communications Commission. With fines exceeding $2,5000,000 he moved his broadcasts off the public airways to private subscription services.

His books *Private Parts* and *Miss America* have been number one on the *New York Times* bestseller list. He frequently describes farts and farting on his programs and has popularized his superhero character of Fartman.

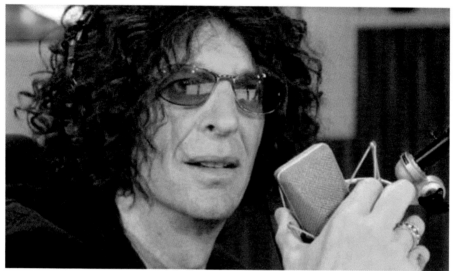

greginhollywood.com/howard-stern

Famous Quotations:

"Most of the things I do are misunderstood. Hey, after all, being misunderstood is the fate of all true geniuses, is it not?"

"Why be uptight about bowel movements and sex? We all have sex. We all have penises -- except for those of us who have vaginas."

"I'm sickened by all religions. Religion has divided people. I don't think there's any difference between the pope wearing a large hat and parading around with a smoking purse and an African painting his face white and praying to a rock."

"I love America. I love our freedom. And nowhere could a guy like me, a schlub like me have success with -- where would I get this freedom of speech? They don't allow this anywhere."

Melina Marchetta

Melina Marchetta (1965-) is an Australian award winning author whose books are especially popular with young adult readers.

Saving Francesca
"These guys fart a lot as well. I'm not saying that girls don't. We just aren't as passionate about them. The smell is sometimes overwhelming and I want to gag. They don't just limit these attacks to the classroom-they can come at you from anywhere around the school. The corridor, the stairwell, the canteen line. There's

one area we call Fart Corridor because it belongs to the Year Eights and Nines, who are the biggest perpetrators. They make no apologies and feel no embarrassment. If a girl did one at St. Stella's she'd be an outcast for the rest of her natural life. Here, it's a badge of honor."

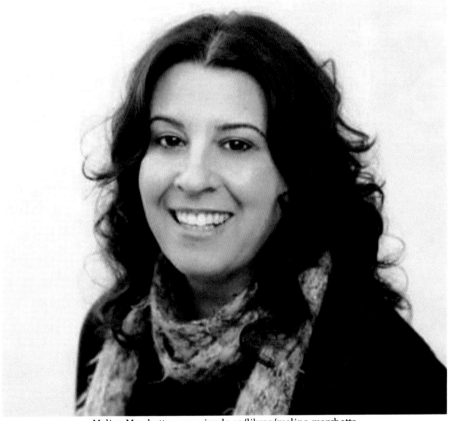

Melina Marchetta www.circulo.es/libros/melina-marchetta

Famous Quotations:

"There are worse things than a lie and there are better things than the truth!"
"Your problems are out there. But they're small. They only grow out of proportion when they climb inside your head."
"I'm not interested in those who do me wrong. There's not enough time in the day for them."
"I can't believe I said it out loud. The truth doesn't set you free, you know. It makes you feel awkward and embarrassed and defenseless and red in the face and horrified and petrified and vulnerable. But free? I don't feel free. I feel like shit."

Children's Books

There has been a figurative explosion in the number of children's books on farts and other bodily functions. One of the early pioneering volumes was *Good Families Don't* by popular Canadian children book authors Robert Munsch and Alan Daniel. The clever, respectful, and witty volume was accepted for publication by Doubleday Canada but only on the condition that the word fart was dropped from the title.

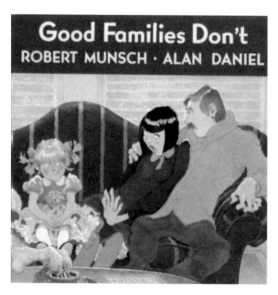

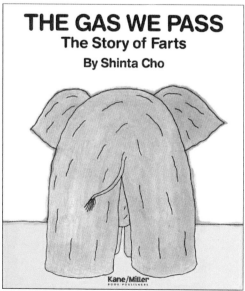

Since this occurred in the 1980's the word fart has reentered the mainstream vocabulary and entertaining and informative children's books with the word fart in the title have prominent window display. *The Gas We Pass: The Story of Farts* by Shinta Cho has become a children's bestseller.

Another in the Everyone Poops series, this book by Shinta Cho is "both informative and blunt," said Publishers Weekly. "The book provides young readers with solid facts as well as plenty to snicker about."

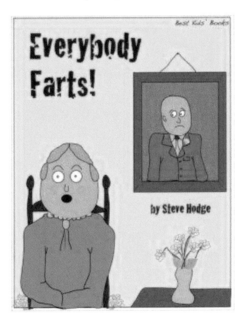

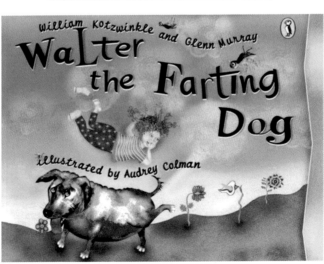

In 2004, a former school board trustee in Wisconsin was so upset over the word "fart" in this story about an old, fat dog with incurable flatulence that he wanted the book banned from the state's school system. The book, *Walter the Farting Dog* mentions the word fart or farting 24 times. His efforts, and others at libraries and school systems across the country were unsuccessful.

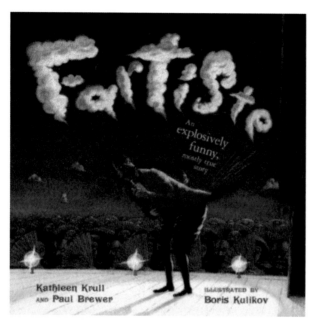

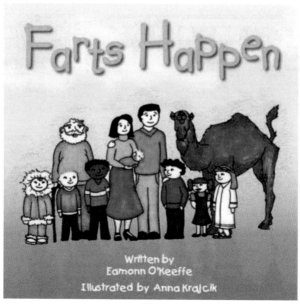

National Post:

All of the librarians "strongly defended" the place of scatologically themed books in the public library system (hey, even Beowulf and Shakespeare included references to feces). More than half said the "intellectual freedom rights" of children to have access to books they enjoy was important. Many said they used such books as Walter the Farting Dog to encourage boys to read, in light of troubling literacy data that shows boys don't enjoy tucking into a book like girls do.

"One of the main reasons librarians defended these books was they felt children [when they start to understand stories] have just gone through a very difficult stage right after potty training — it's been the entire focus of the child's life and focus of much of the interaction between parent and child," Ms. Curry said. "But as soon as the child is potty trained, then all of a sudden you're not supposed to talk about it. A child yelling in the library, 'Mommy, mom I need to poo poo' is met with a shhhh…. That's why kids are enjoying this. They're trying to figure out what is taboo and what isn't."

Having a book in the library that celebrates this taboo is "something they find really funny" because they know they're not supposed to exclaim the words out loud, Ms. Curry said. It also helps make children more aware of their bodies, able to identify their various parts and not be ashamed, she added.

Even still, librarians expressed frustration with parents who "believed that public library children's collections should contain just 'the best literature,' " Ms. Curry's paper reads. "Immensely popular books like Captain Underpants were deemed by these parents to be a waste of taxpayer dollars and more appropriate for low-class bookstores."

Librarians also felt parents wanted to censor the books because they brought out "animalistic" tendencies in their children instead of "higher moral thoughts of a well-behaved child."

"The librarians who had lots of experience as children's librarians did mention that they felt disapproval of this type of information had decreased considerably over the years," Ms. Curry said. "Part of the reason for that is this material is discussed much more openly in the general media."

Oprah's clinician-in-residence Dr. Oz openly talks about poop, and such reality TV shows as Fear Factor and Survivor are full of people being forced to eat gross things, she said.

And in the two decades since Canadian publisher Doubleday told children's author Robert Munsch he could not put the word "Fart" on the cover of his book

Good Families Don't..., publishers have rushed to cash in on the "fashion of farting."

Of course, some librarians themselves were grossed out by a number of the scatological books, Ms. Curry found, also noting that a surprising number of these were in translation (the book Everybody Poops is translated from Japanese; The Little Mole Who Knew It Was None of His Business was originally penned in German).

At the end of the day, most were just happy to get a book into children's hands, said Ms. Curry, who says her research into scatological children's books provides a broader context for the study of censorship in libraries across Canada.

A Norwegian author and musician, Jo Nesbø has sold more than one and a half million copies of his novels in Norway alone. Nesbø is considered to be a leading crime and thriller novelist in Europe. His books have been translated into more than 40 languages for a worldwide readership.

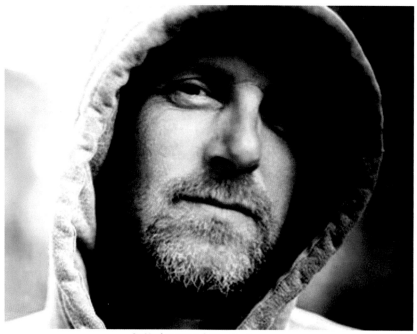

Jo Nesbø www.famousauthors.org

The *Doktor Proktor* series by Jo Nesbø was created for children. The first book of the series, *Doctor Proctor's Fart Powder* was released in 2007 followed by *Doctor Proctor's Fart Powder: Bubble in the Bathtub* in 2008. The third book of the series, *Doctor Proctor and the Destruction of the World* was published in 2010.

IX. Colloquialism, Idiom, & Synonym of Fart

The word fart is one of the oldest words in the English language. One of the most important dictionaries in the long history of the language is Samuel Johnson's *A Dictionary of the English Language* published in 1755. An important innovation in his dictionary was the use of quotations from literature to illustrate the usage of the word defined.

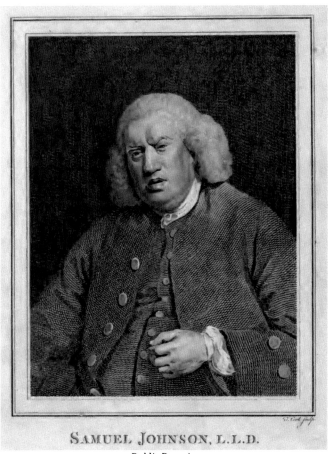

SAMUEL JOHNSON, L.L.D.

Public Domain

The word fart is proper English, and was in use for hundreds of years, before relatively recent polite and civil society considered it taboo. Without an alternative word, euphemisms were created and used. The number of terms that were synonymous with fart numbers in the many hundreds. The partial list that follows gives a good approximation of the wide variety of colorful alternatives.

The origins of these phrases, and their acceptance into the cultural lexicon, are often obscured. Sometimes new words are added simply by an author creatively using a newly invented word in a literary work. I am fond of a new word coined by David Gilmour, an entrepreneur and philanthropist. He described a word that combines the sense of anticipation and subsequent disappointment, when the experience is not as satisfying as expected. The word he crated 'anticipointment' is a portmanteau that should stand the test of time.

I am tempted to add to new words to the lexicon as well. I am using the author's prerogative to place the words in print below, and although I have not heard them elsewhere before someone may well have created them before me. The first word is fartigenic, or its alternative, fartogenic. Fartigenic is a portmanteau combining the word fart with the Latin root suffix -genic of genesis and creation fame. The word describes a substance, which induces the creation of a fart. Refried beans and chili con carne would be good examples of fartigenic foods.

My second word creation choice would be related to the common phrase stomach flu when used to describe a viral gastroenteritis with diarrhea and farting. We often use the term flu when describing a viral illness even though in is not a true influenza virus. I am taking poetic liberty to borrow the influenza root word to describe a stomach flu as 'inflatuenza'.

My third and final word would be an alternative word for bloating or distention. As one could consider this condition to be caused by the retention and delay of the necessary intestinal gas passage, I suggest the word 'gastipated'. Okay, so maybe that word will not stand the test of time, and I should cease my word mining activities while I still have you as a reader.

What follows are the colloquialisms, idioms, and synonyms, that for better or for worse, are part of the lexicon.

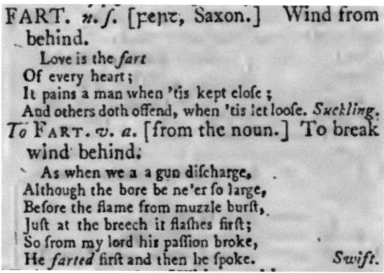

FART. *n. ʃ.* [ꝼeꞃꞇ, Saxon.] Wind from behind.

    Love is the *fart*
Of every heart;
It pains a man when 'tis kept clofe;
And others doth offend, when 'tis let loofe. *Suckling.*
To FART. *v. a.* [from the noun.] To break wind behind.

  As when we a a gun difcharge,
Although the bore be ne'er fo large,
Before the flame from muzzle burft,
Juft at the breech it flafhes firft;
So from my lord his paffion broke,
He *farted* firft and then he fpoke.   *Swift.*

A bit more choke and you would have started – an Australian phrase often addressed to the person responsible for an audible fart

Afflatus – Although it contains the word flatus this word has nothing to do with a fart. Flatus is Latin for a blowing, breathing, or a wind. Afflatus is a word first used by Cicero in his volume *De Natura Deorum* (*The Nature of the Gods*). In his book it is used as a phrase for a sudden rush of unexpected breath, a fresh inspiration. The word inspiration is derived from inspire, to breath as well as to have a creative thought or new idea. Afflatus thus can mean a divine inspiration. The only way to associate it with a fart is to consider it to be the exact opposite of a brain fart .

After thunder comes the rain – Phrase used when fart is passed just before urinating.

Air bagel – Fart

Air biscuit – Fart

Anal acoustics - Fart

Anal ahem - Fart

Anal audio - Fart

Anal salute - Fart

Anal volcano - Fart

Aqua fart - An underwater fart bubble, usually seen in the bathtub or swimming pool. The only way to clearly see an otherwise invisible fart.

Arse blast - Fart

Artsy Fartsy – Presented as art and culture but just as likely to be seen as pretentious, eccentric, eclectic, and unworthy of sophisticated cultural approval.

As much chance as a fart in a thunderstorm, windstorm, blizzard, hurricane, tornado, gale, etcetera - Means having no chance at all.

Ass blaster - Fart

Ass biscuit - Fart

Ass thunder - Fart

Ass whistle - Fart

Brain fart – Mental lapse, which usually results in an error while doing a repetitive activity.

Backdoor breeze - Fart

Backfire - Fart

Barking spiders - Fart

Bean blower - Fart

Blast off - Fart

Blowing a Raspberry (or Strawberry) – Imitating the sound of a fart by exhaling through pursed lips, usually as a sign of derision. Also known as a Bronx cheer.

Blowing the butt bugle - Fart

Blowing you a kiss - Fart

Bomber - Fart

Bottom blast - Fart

Bottom burp - Fart

Break wind - Fart

Breath of fresh air - Fart
Bronx cheer - Imitating the sound of a fart by exhaling through pursed lips, usually as a sign of derision. Also known as a Blowing a Raspberry or Strawberry.
Brown horn brass choir - Fart
Brown thunder - Fart
Bun shaker - Fart
Burnin' rubber - Fart
Buster - Fart
Busting ass - Fart
Butt bleat - Fart
Butt burp - Fart
Butt percussion - Fart
Butt trumpet - Fart
Butt tuba - Fart
Buttock bassoon - Fart
Cheek flapper - Fart
Cheesin' - Fart
Colonic calliope - Fart
Crack a rat - Fart
Crack one off - Fart
Crack splitters - Fart
Crop dusting - Farting while passing seated bystanders
Crowd splitter - Fart
Cut a stinker - Fart
Cut loose - Fart
Cut the cheese - Fart
Cut the wind - Fart
Death breath - Fart
Deflate - Fart
Drop a barking spider - Fart
Drop a bomb - Fart
Drop ass - Fart
Dutch oven – Farting under the blankets while in bed, then covering up your bedmate to share the aroma.
Empty my tank - Fart
Eproctophilia – A fart fetish, the receiving of sexual pleasure and arousal from the fart of another. The author James Joyce (see separate entry) describes this fetish in letters published after his death.
Exploding bottom - Fart
Exterminate - Fart
Farst – Descriptive of a fast fart

Fart – (Foreign languages) – Unrelated to the English usage of the word, in the German and Scandinavian languages the word means speed, often used in speeding or speed control zones signs. in Danish a *fartcertifikate* means a trade certificate. In Norwegian a *fart plan* means a schedule. The Norwegian phrase *stå på fartin* pronounced as stop-a –fartin means ready to leave. Likewise the phrase *farts måler* pronounced as fart smeller refers to a speedometer. In Swedish a speed bump is called a *farthinder*. *Fartlek* is speed training by running at alternate intervals of fast and slow paces.. Likewise if you travel on a Scandinavian marine vessel you may see the control of engine speed labeled as *half fart* and *full fart* for half speed and full speed respectively. Fart kontrol zones are speed zones. In Germany a similar word *fahrt* means a journey, trip, tour, or passage. It is often seen in signs that say e*infahrt* (sounds like in-fart) and *ausfahrt* (sounds like out-fart) denoting entrance and exit respectively. In Spanish and Portuguese *fart* means an excess of anything, especially a food. One of the richest deserts they offer is called a *farte*, which means a fruit tarte in Spain and usually a sugar almond or cream cake in Portugal. In Italy the word *farto* means mattress. In Hungarian *fartaj* means buttocks. In Poland if you want to buy a popular candy bar with a name that that means lucky you will be looking for a *Fart* bar.

Fartalito - Word for a small fart combining English and Spanish (Spanglish)
Fartable farter – An individual who can fart on command
Fart about – Waste time on silly or unnecessary activities
Fart absorption ratio – Humorous descriptive of the quantity of farts that a material can absorb and retain before the trapped gas escapes. Usually used to describe furniture such as a chair, sofa, ottoman, cushions, mattress, but can also be applied to rugs, carpets, clothing, etcetera.
Fart ache – Descriptive of a fart so potent that exposure to the fumes gives a headache. May also be used to describe pain after farting with anorectal disease such as fissures, abscess, fistula, hemorrhoids, and after delivery or surgery.
Fartachoo – A fart and sneeze occurring simultaneously
Fartacious – Ability to produce copious farts, either by volume or frequency.
Fartacrite – An individual who is hypocritical about farts, considering the farts of others as objectionable while their own farts are perfectly acceptable.
Fart addict – One who is obsessed with farting, usually used to describe an individual who produces farts in prodigious frequency and quantity.
Fartage - (French) Waxing of cross-country skis, unrelated to fart.
Fart against thunder – The fart equivalent of urinating (pissing) into the wind.
Fartagious – Contagious farting, often noted in preadolescent males.
Fartaholic – An individual who is described as being addicted to farting, often used to describe a husband.
Fart alarm – When the need to fart is misinterpreted as the need to defecate. Also when a baby's diaper is changed assuming a bowel movement occurred, only to find the diaper is empty as it was just a fart.
Fartalicious – A particularly attractive fart, either by acoustics, aroma, or quantity. Also may be used as a sarcastic compliment denoting that the taste of a food or drink was offensive.
Fart amnesty – A zone where unhindered farting is allowed without criticism or limitation. The zone is usually defined by the significant other, and may be in a remote location and different time zone.
Fart and dart – An individual who release a fart and quickly departs to let others

experience their fart. Also known as fart and run.

Fart and flee – A practical joke, often executed spontaneously on releasing a fart in a crowded public place. The person immediately behind you is left standing in the aromatic wake of your fart, is assumed to be the culprit, and is the recipient of abhorrent glares from others.

Fart angels – Actively moving arms and legs in the same fashion as one makes snow angels by lying down in the snow. The activity is done in the standing mode to help circulate the air in the hope of dissipating the smell.

Fartanoid – A frantic sense of insecurity that an impending fart may allow the release of bowel contents.

Fartapalooza – A spasm of frequent, voluminous, and typically audacious farts over a short period of time. More often occurs following ingestion of a fart inducing meal, such as refried beans.

Fart app – An application for mobile phones and other electronic devices that reproduces sounds that imitate the various acoustic forms of the art of the fart.

Fart around – Waste time on silly or unnecessary activities

Fart arpeggio – A fart that changes tone at least twice so that three or more notes are produced during its course. A master of this technique was Joseph Pujol, known as Le Pétomane, during his performance career on the Moulin Rouge in Paris.

Fartarrhea – Similar to shart as a combination of shit and fart, but with diarrhea and fart. The fart often releases a mist of liquid feces, which soil the underwear or clothing if not released while on a toilet.

Fart arse – (British) To be stupid, farting or mucking around.

Fart art – Euphemism for abstract art appearance of soiling of underwear upon passing a particularly powerful fart that carried some organic fecal matter, mucus, or moisture. More common with a bout of dysentery or diarrhea.

Fart ass – Similar to smart-ass

Fart attack – Condition of pain related to intestinal gas, including intestinal gas in the pre-fart stage of bloating and distension. Play on words with similarity to heart attack, Unfortunately symptoms that suggest intestinal gas discomfort (fart attack) may actually be due to a heart condition (heart attack) and delay urgently needed medical care. In this situation a misdiagnosed fart/heart attack can be a true life threatening condition.

Fart baby – Descriptive term for abdominal bloating from intestinal gas, more noticeable in young thin women who develop visible distension that gives the impression of an early pregnancy.

Fart bag – A plastic or paper bag used to capture and seal in a fart, to be subsequently opened in the face of an unsuspecting victim.

Fart bellows – Farting under a blanket while in bed, and then trying to clear the fart by using the blanket as a bellow. The opposite of a Dutch oven, where the goal is to trap the fart under the blanket.

Fart blanche – To be given carte blanche to fart at will under the blanket or other locations.

Fart box – A euphemism for anus, rectum, and rectal cavity.

Fart brain – Used similarly to airhead, suggesting that farts rather than brains reside in the skull

Fart breath – Foul smelling breath

Fart bride – A woman who was very discrete about bodily functions, especially farts, before marriage, but loses all inhibitions after marriage.

Fart bubble – An underwater fart bubble, usually seen in the bathtub or swimming pool. The only way to clearly see an otherwise invisible fart.

Fart catcher – Nickname given to horsemen seated immediately behind the horses pulling a carriage. Also used to describe assistants and servants who walk a few paces behind their superior.

Fart buddy – A friend who is close enough that farting in their presence does not lead to any offense, and may contribute to an open farting atmosphere.

Fart burn – The burning rectal or anal sensation after extensive diarrhea and farting. Also may be experienced after eating hotly spiced foods.

Fart camouflage – Also known as fart camo. Making noise by an activity to hide the sound of a fart. The goal is to create a distraction to allow the noisy passage of a fart to go undetected. Using an air freshener, perfume, or other strong aroma may be used in an attempt to mask the smell. Opening windows and doors with the excuse that it is too warm is often used as a fart camouflage maneuver.

Fart candy – Candy that induces farting by having a high content of non-absorbable sugars. Dietetic candies often have this property.

Fart door - Colloquial term for anus.

Farter – A person who procrastinates by farting around. (British) Slang term for anus, also a sleeping bag which is warmed by farts.

Farterbox – (Irish) Slang for anus

Fartface – Facial expression that gives the impression that the wearer is smelling a noxious fart. Also slang for an idiot or stupid person.

Fart factory – Slang for anus, also to describe a frequent or voluminous farter.

Fart fetish – Formally known as eproctophilia, the receiving of sexual pleasure and arousal from the fart of another. The author James Joyce (see separate entry) describes this fetish in letters published after his death.

Farther, Farthest, Farthermost – These words denote greater distance from an object, an are unrelated to the word fart that is contained within their spelling. The only way they may be tied to the word fart is in vocabulary games like Scrabble, Boggle, and others where additional points may be gained by adding letters to a core word.

Fart higher than your ass – Arrogant and pretentious, translation of original phrase from the French *péter plus haut que son cul.*

Farthing – British coin currency with a nominal value. Benjamin Franklin uses the nominal currency as a double entendre at the end of his proposal to the Royal Academy of Brussels to create an award for an additive that word give farts a pleasant smell (see entry under Benjamin Franklin).

Farthingale – A hoop like structure worn under the skirt by women in the late 16th and early 17th centuries to give it the shape of a bell or cone. Originally introduced at the Spanish court it subsequently became popular fashion in Tudor England. Although the shape and structure may have been helpful to muffle the sound and contain the aroma of a fart, there is no evidence that the name was related to the word fart. One theory behind the development of the farthingale was to hide a pregnancy that may have resulted from illicit relationships.

Fart in a bottle – Description of restless movement suggestive of agitation or being flustered.

Fart in a thunderstorm or windstorm – Figure of speech suggesting the event is unnoticed or unidentifiable because of background activity. When in the phrase as much chance as a fart in a thunderstorm, windstorm, blizzard, hurricane, tornado, gale, etc. it means having no chance at all.

Farting clapper - Anus, or more pejorative asshole.

Farting fanny – Nickname given to heavy German artillery guns used during World War I

Farting shot – An action designed to show contempt.

Farting through silk – financially affluent, able to afford luxuries

Fart lighting – Ignition of flammable gas (methane and/or hydrogen) released in some farts. Serious injury and burns have resulted from this activity, most often seen in adolescent males.

Fartman – A fictional superhero popularized by television and radio personality Howard Stern (see separate entry).

Fart monkey – Term of endearment, usually for a pet such as a dog or cat that farts whenever it needs to. The fart monkey can also serve as fart camouflage and be designated as the source of an errant fart.

Fart sucker – A parasite or toady willing to do whatever it takes to curry favor. Analogous to ass kisser, brown-nose equivalent. Interesting tie in to French slang for criminal suspect. The French pronounce suspect as soos-pay, the same way they would pronounce the words *sucé pet*, which translates literally as fart sucker. The French authorities can use the double entendre to express their dislike of a suspect without being chastised.

Fart time – Describes employed hours per week that fall between full-time and part-time employment. Usually defined as between 21 and 35 hours of work time per week.

Fire a stink torpedo - Fart

Fire the retro-rocket - Fart

Firing scud missiles - Fart

Fizzler - Fart

Flamethrower - Fart

Flamer - Fart

Flapper - Fart

Flatulate - Fart

Flatulence - Fart

Flatus - Fart

Flipper - Fart

Float an air biscuit - Fart

Floof - Fart

Fluffy - Fart

Fog slicer - Fart
Fowl howl - Fart
Fragrant fuzzy - Fart
Free-floating anal vapors - Fart
Free Jacuzzi - Fart
Freep - Fart
Frequency Actuated Rectal Tremor - Fart
Fumigate - Fart
Funky rollers - Fart
Gas attack - Fart
Gas blaster - Fart
Gas from the ass - Fart
Gas master - Fart
Gaseous intestinal by-products – Fart
Ghost turd - Fart
Grandpa - Fart
Gravy pants - Fart
Great brown cloud - Fart
Heinus anus - Fart
Hole flappage - Fart
Hole flapper - Fart
Honk - Fart
HUMrrhoids - Fart
Hydrogen bomb - Fart
Ignition - Fart
Insane in the methane - Fart
Invert a burp - Fart
Jet propulsion - Fart
Joan of Fart – Artful nickname for a female who has farted audibly or aromatically.
Jockey burner - Fart
Jumping guts - Fart
Just calling your name - Fart
Just keeping warm - Fart
Just the noise - Fart
Kaboom - Fart
K-Fart - Fart
Kill the canary - Fart
Lay a wind loaf - Fart
Lay an air biscuit - Fart
Leave a gas trap - Fart
Let a beefer - Fart
Let a brewer's fart – To have diarrhea.
Let each little bean be heard - Fart
Let one fly - Fart
Let one go - Fart
Let the beans out - Fart

Lethal cloud - Fart
Letting one rip - Fart
Lingerer - Fart
Made a gas blast – Fart
Make a stink - Fart
Make a trumpet of one's ass – Fart
Mating call of the barking spider - Fart
Meteor – Fart
Methane bomb - Fart
Methane production experiment - Fart
Moon gas - Fart
Mud duck - Fart
Must be a sewer around - Fart
Nose death - Fart
Odor bubble - Fart
Odorama - Fart
Old fart – An old man, a person in authority very set in their ways, inflexible.
One-man jazz band - Fart
One-gun salute - Fart
Painting the elevator - Fart
Pant stainer - Fart
Panty burp - Fart
Parp - Fart
Party in your pants - Fart
Pass gas - Fart
Pass wind - Fart
Pet – Fart (French) The diminutive for fart in the French language. It makes the written English use of pet shop, pet food, love of pets, etc. an interesting translation. The pronunciation is different however, as pet is pronounced as pay in French
Pissed as a fart – Very drunk (British & Australian)
Play the tuba - Fart
Playing the trouser tuba - Fart
Plotcher (aka a wet one) – Fart
Poof - Fart
Poop gas - Fart
Poot - Fart
Pootie – Fart
Pop - Fart
Pop a fluffy - Fart
Preventing spontaneous human combustion – Fart
Puff, the magic dragon - Fart
Quack - Fart
Raspberry (Razz) - Slang for *'blowing a raspberry or strawberry'*, imitating the sound of a fart by exhaling through pursed lips, usually as a sign of derision. Also known as a Bronx cheer.

Rebuild the ozone layer one poof at a time - Fart
Rectal honk - Fart
Rectal shout - Fart
Rectal tremor - Fart
Release a squeaker - Fart
Release an ass biscuit - Fart
Release gas - Fart
Rep - Fart
Rimshot - Fart
Rip ass - Fart
Rip one - Fart
Ripple fart - Fart
Roast the Jockeys - Fart
Rotting vegetation - Fart
Royal fart – A fart of unusual distinction.
Safety - Fart
Salute your shorts - Fart
SAS (silent and scentless) – Fart
SBD (silent but deadly) – Fart
Set off an SBD - Fart
Shart – Fart passage that allows the escape of fecal material. The word shart is a portmanteau of shit and fart.
Shit fumes - Fart
Shit honker - Fart
Shit vapor - Fart
Shoot the cannon - Fart
Shoppin' at Wal-Fart - Fart
Silent and scentless (SAS) – Fart
Silent but deadly (SBD) – Fart
Singe the carpet - Fart
Singing the anal anthem - Fart
Sounding the sphincter scale - Fart
Sound of a barking spider - Fart
Sound of a wompus cat - Fart
Sparrow-fart - Denotes the earliest of daylight, early dawn, sunrise, sunup, first light of day.
Sphincter song - Fart
Spit a brick - Fart
Squeak one out - Fart
Squeaker - Fart
Steamer - Fart
Step on a duck - Fart
Step on a frog - Fart
Stink bomb - Fart
Stink burger - Fart

Strangling the stank monkey - Fart
Strawberry - Slang for imitating the sound of a fart by exhaling through pursed lips, usually as a sign of derision. Also known as a Bronx cheer.
Stress release - Fart
Tail wind - Fart
The colonic calliope - Fart
The dog did it - Fart
The F bomb - Fart
The gluteal tuba - Fart
The Sound and the Fury - Fart
The stink's gone into the fabric - Fart
The third state of matter - Fart
The toothless one speaks - Fart
Thunder pants - Fart
Thunderspray - Fart
Toilet tune - Fart
Toot - Fart
Toot your own horn - Fart
Trelblow - Fart
Triple flutter blast - Fart
Trouser cough - Fart
Trouser trumpet - Fart
Turd honking - Fart
Turd hooties - Fart
Turn on the air conditioning in the colon - Fart
Uncorked symphony - Fart
Under burp - Fart
Venting one - Fart
Wet one - Fart
What the dog did - Fart
Who Cut the Cheese - Fart
Wrong way burping - Fart
Zinger – Fart

X. Fart in Foreign Languages

American Sign Language:

The non-dominant hand is an "A" or an "S" handshape. The dominant hand is a bent hand and is held so that the fingers are underneath the pinkie side of the non-dominant "fist." The dominant hand "unbends" and bends one time as if showing gas escaping. Here is a "one handed" version of fart, both versions are widely used. You start by opening up the pinkie, and then the ring and middle finger. The index finger stays curled up. Then you reverse and close the middle, then ring, then pinkie fingers. For comic effect or emphasis you can puff one cheek and force a bit of air through your lips at the corner of your mouth.

Afrikaans: fart
Albanian: pordhÃ«, pjerdh; pordhë, hajvan, pjerdh
Arabic: ضرطة‎, ضرطنفخة‎, ha ridge
Armenian: fart, basz toe
Avestan: pərəδaiti
Azerbaijani: osurmaq
Basque: fart
Belarusian: Ð¿ÐµÑ€Ð´ÐµÑ‚,ÑŒ
Bulgaria: fart Флатуленция, пръдня
Catalan: pet, *colloq* pet, *colloq* torracollons, *colloq* tirar-se un pet, fer-se un pet
Chinese (Simplified): 屁, 放屁 屁 fom pee/ pie Chee

Chinese (Traditional): 屁, 放屁 屁 fom pee/ pie Chee
Croatian: prdnuti, vjetar, prdac, ispuštati vjetrove, prditi
Czech: prd
Danish: prut
Dutch: wind laten, winderigheid, een wind laten, een scheet laten, (slang) scheet (slang)
Esperanto: furzi, furzo
Estonian: pieru
Farsi: gooz bede, گوز ، گوزیدن‎
Filipino: umut-ot, kabag-gas oh mo toot ka
Finnish: pieru
French: péter, pet, dis gas, péter (argot); lâcher une vesse; vesser pet (argot), vesse, merdeux
Galician: peidar
Georgian: fart
German: furz, flatulenz, fuhren sie gas, furzen, sich mit jedem dreck abgeben (Umgangsprache), scheißer (slang)
Greek: πέρδομαι (perdomai), Î°Î»Î±Î½Î½Î¹Î¬, κλάνω, πέρδομαι κλανιά, πορδή
Haitian Creole: fart
Hebrew: להפליץ" ,"לתקוע נאד" "סלנג (נפיחה "באד) "סלנג")
Hindi: ☐☐☐☐☐

Hmong: tso paus, tawb paus
Hungarian: fing, fingik, szellentés
Icelandic: rÃ¦fill
Ilokano: uttot
Indonesian: kentut
Irish: fart
Italian: fart, flatulenza, pass il gas, scoreggiare scoreggio, peto
Japanese: おなら, 屁, おならをする, 屁をこく（俗語） おなら, 屁（俗語）
Korean: 방귀뀌다, bung koo
Latin: pēdĕre
Latvian: fart
Lithuanian: bezdalius
Macedonia: Ð¿Ñ€Ð´ÐµÐ¶
Malay: kentut
Maltese: fart
Norwegian: fart
Persian: گوز، گوزیدن, گوز gooz bede
Philippine: kabag-gas, oh mo toot ka, umut-ot,
Polish: bpierd, pierdzieÄ‡, gazy jelitowe, parvee etra, vi pierdzieć, pierdnięcie, pierdnąć
Portugese: peidar, pedo, flatulência, soltar um pum (gíria) peido,
Romanian: bÄƒÅŸi, flatulenţă, gaze (vulgar), vint, a da vinturi,

Russian: пердеть (perdet'), издавать громкий треск, пукнуть громкий треск при выходе газов из организма, непристойный звук; пукание; старик зря терять время Ð¿ÐµÑ€Ð´ÐµÑ‚ÑŒ, метеоризм, puk nee
The Russian words for fart include *perdyozh* (first act of breaking wind), *perdun* (perpetrator and outcome), *perdil'nik* (place from where it comes), *Perun* (ancient God of wind), *bzdun* (silent fart), *bzdyukha* (silent fart as well as a stupid jerk). Some of the Russian verbs for the action of farting are particularly colorful. *Perdet'* (to fart with or without sound), *bzdet'* (to fart silently), *pereperdet* (to fart repeatedly), and my favorite word *nabzdet'sya* (ton fart silently to one's complete and utter satisfaction!).

Sanskrit: pardate
Serbian: Ð¿Ñ€Ð´Ð½ÑƒÑ‚Ð¸
Slovak: prd
Slovenian: prdec
Somali: doughso
Spanish: pedo, tirarse un pedo (familismo), peo, pasar gasses, peer, ventosear, ventoseo, cuesco
Swahili: fart, kyfoosi
Swedish: fart, fjärt , flatulens, prutta, fjärta (slang) prutt, fjärt (slang)
Tagalog (Philippine): kabag-gas, oh mo toot ka, umut-ot,
Taiwanese: 放屁 屁 funkee-pass gas

Thai: ตด, ฟาท, ลมตด (ผายลม),ตด,การผายลม,บตก,ผายลม
Turkish: osuruk, ul cer, osurmak, gaz yapmak osuruk, yellenme
Urdu: گوز پاد-پھسکي-باؤ-گوز پادنا-پاد يا پھسکي مارنا-باؤ سڑنا
Vietnamese: đánh rắm, trung tiện, dit, danh từ, đùi 0 rắm,
nội động từ, chùi gháu
Visayan: otot
Welsh: basio gwynt
Yiddish: פֿאַרצן

XI. Afterword

Artsy Fartsy, Cultural History of the Fart is a fascinating and factually correct review of the common fart through human culture and history. It has a companion volume: ***To 'Air' is Human, Everything You Ever Wanted to Know About Intestinal Gas, which*** uniquely informative, entertaining, and well-illustrated. It covers everything you ever wanted to know about the fart, burp, and bloat but were too embarrassed to ask. Intestinal gas has been produced and released by virtually every human who has ever lived, yet very few people have been provided with the knowledge that can offer comfort and relief.

This volume is overflowing with practical information, fascinating facts, surprising trivia, and tasteful humorous insight about this universal phenomenon. Extensive knowledge about the physiology and science of the digestive process and intestinal gas is clearly explained. The knowledge gained will contribute to your enhanced health and comfort, and sharing this wisdom with others can leave a lasting impression on friends and family.

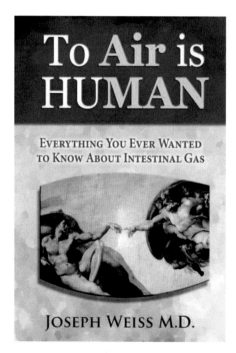

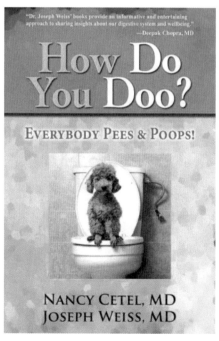

How Do You Doo? Everybody Pees & Poops! A delightfully informative, entertaining, and colorfully illustrated volume with valuable practical insights on toilet training. Tasteful color photographs of animals answering the call of nature allows the child to understand that everybody does it! Additional informative relevant content to entertain the adult while the child is 'on the potty' is included.

The Scoop on Poop! Flush with Knowledge is a uniquely informative tastefully entertaining, and well-illustrated volume that is full of it! The 'it' being a comprehensive and knowledgeable overview of all topics related to the remains of the digestive process. Whether you call it poop, feces, excrement, manure, dung, or the hundred plus other euphemisms, shit happens, and it happens a lot! Tens of billions of pounds and kilograms of it or deposited every day by while diversity of animal and microbial life. Humans alone contribute over three billion pounds a day, and only a small percentage of that is treated by a sewage system

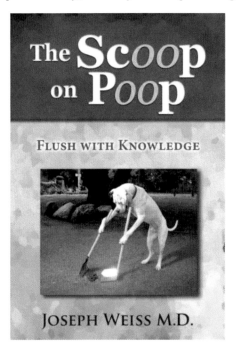 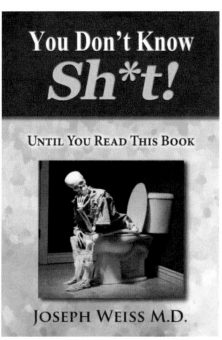

The identical content of The Scoop on Poop has been provocatively and cheekily retitled as ***You Don't Know Sh*t! Until You Read This Book.*** This volume is an informative, entertaining and colorfully illustrated fountain of knowledge that is full of valuable information, including eccentricities and peculiarities, about the remains of the digestive process. Although this end result is politely described as feces or excrement, it is more commonly known by one of oldest words in the English language, shit. The book covers everything you ever wanted to know about this subject. Whether you disdain it, or appreciate it, it is part of the human (and animal) experience. The purpose of this volume is to share rarely discussed but very important knowledge about poop. The information ranges from the potentially life-saving to the sidesplitting descriptions of the eccentricities and peculiarities of human behavior on the subject matter. The wealth of information and trivia can sustain a long social conversation, or cut it short abruptly!

AirVeda: Ancient & New Medical Wisdom, Digestion & Gas covers the remarkable advances in the understanding of digestive health and wellness. New information about the critical role of genomics, epigenetics, the gut microbiome, and the gut-brain-microbiome-diet axis are opening new avenues to optimal whole body health and wellness. An appreciation of the ancient wisdom of Ayurveda and other disciplines shows that they had advanced insights into the nature of the human body and the holistic approach. Although intestinal gas, basic bodily functions, and feces have been topics culturally suppressed, knowledge and understanding are needed to achieve and maintain optimal health. This volume, and others in the series, provide an informative and entertaining in depth look at the amazing world of human health and digestion.

"Ayurveda is a 5,000 year old system of natural healing that reminds us that health is the balanced and dynamic integration between our environment, body, mind and spirit. In Dr. Joseph Weiss' book, AirVeda, he provides an informative and entertaining approach to sharing insights about our digestive system and wellbeing by applying the ancient wisdom of Ayurveda to everyday life." **Deepak Chopra, MD**

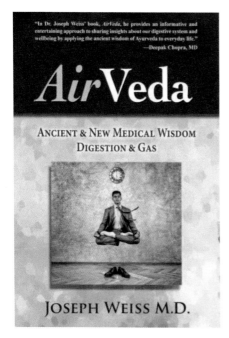
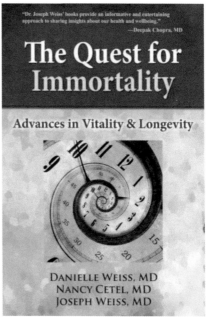

The Quest for Immortality, Advances in Vitality & Longevity provides an informative and enlightening overview of the remarkable advances in science and medicine that are dramatically enhancing human health and lifespan. The volume is written in clear, understandable, and engaging language with striking colorful illustrations. From groundbreaking nanotechnology to genomics and stem cells, the secrets of vitality and longevity are being uncovered along with more traditional advances and practical insights into disease prevention and health enhancement.

An even more comprehensive yet entertaining series are the extensive volumes of *Digestive Health & Disease, An Illustrated Encyclopedia of Everything You Ever Wanted To Know About Digestion & Nutrition*. These volumes are a uniquely informative, entertaining, and lavishly illustrated compendium of alimentary knowledge and eccentricities. It covers everything you ever wanted to know about digestion and nutrition in health and disease. Volumes One through Five are available on Amazon.com.

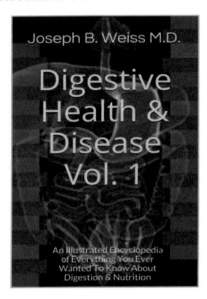 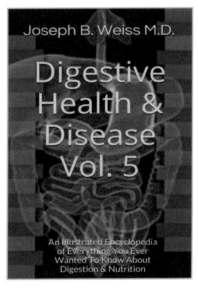

Organized as a reader friendly encyclopedia, the volumes cover over two thousand five hundred subject topics. Each volume may be utilized as an independent fully contained resource for the subjects it covers. The extensive size and scope of the series allows topics to be included that are rarely discussed in other books in the field and may be of great interest to the curious mind.

Written for the intelligent lay public, the medical and scientific terminology is translated into plain English. Practical and useful information and guidance are the primary goals, but entertaining and interesting information is included wherever possible. Designed for the visual learner as well, the clearly written text is supplemented by excellent photographs, illustrations, and charts. The reader will be informed, entertained, and the beneficiary of their newfound understanding of the universal process of digestion and metabolism that is the basis of all healthy living.

The website www.smartaskbooks.com has a complete list of books and programs by Joseph Weiss, MD, FACP, FACG, AGAF, Clinical Professor of Medicine (Gastroenterology), University of California, San Diego.

XII Index (including Volume One)

Advertising & Marketing Vol. 1
Aerophagia Vol. 1
Afterword 155-158
Alighieri, Dante 28-29
Arabia, Lawrence of Vol. 1
Arabian Nights 26-28
Aristophanes 22-24
Aristotle Vol. 1
Arouet, François-Marie (Voltaire) 55-58
Aubrey, John 48
Auden, W.H. 108-109
Augustine of Hippo (Saint Augustine) Vol. 1
Augustine, Saint Vol. 1
Babylonian Talmud Vol. 1
Balzac, Honoré 65-66
Banks, Iain 130-132
Barth, John 118-119
Baudelaire, Charles Pierre 70
Beardsley, Aubrey Vol. 1
Beavis & Butt-head Vol. 1
Bel-Phegor 21-22
Beckett, Samuel 111-112
Bible Prophets Vol. 1
Blake, William 60-61
Blount, Thomas Vol. 1
Boilly, Louis-Léopold Vol. 1
Bollywood Hindi Movie Vol. 1
Bosch, Hieronymus Vol. 1
Bourke, John Gregory 21, 46, Vol. 1
Brillat-Savarin, Jean Anthelme 59-60
Bruegel the Elder, Pieter Vol. 1
Brooks, Mel Vol. 1
Budweiser Super Bowl Commercial Vol. 1
Burton, Sir Richard Vol. 1
Bush, George W. Vol. 1
Canadian Broadcast Corporation Vol. 1
Canterbury Tales 31-33
Carlin, George 123-126
Cartoonists Vol. 1
Chaucer, Geoffrey 31-33
Children's Book Art Vol. 1
Children's Books 135-139

Chronology of Farts in the Arts Vol. 1
Chronology of Farts in History Vol. 1
Chronology of Farts in Literature Vol. 2
Churchill, Sir Winston Vol. 1
Cicero Vol. 1
Cinematic Arts Vol. 1
Claudius Vol. 1
Clemens, Samuel (Mark Twain) 73-93
Colloquialism, Idiom, & Synonym of Fart 140-151
Commercial, Budweiser Super Bowl Vol. 1
Crepitation Contest Vol. 1
Cromwell, Oliver Vol. 1
Cruikshank, George 47-49
Cushion, Whoopee Vol. 1
Dahl, Roald 109-111
Dalai Lama of Tibet, H.H. the 14th Vol. 1
Dali, Salvador Vol. 1
Dante Alighieri 28-29
De Balzac, Honoré 65-66
Defoe, Daniel 49-50
De Gaulle, Charles Vol. 1
Dent, William Vol. 1
De Plancy, Jacques Collin 64-65
De Verville, Francois Béroalde 40-42
Digestion 7-20
di Lodovico Buonarroti Simoni, Michelangelo Vol. 1
Divine Comedy 28-29
Donne, John 44-45
Earl of Rochester, Lord John Wilmot 50-51
Elagabalus Vol. 1
Elizabeth I, HRH Queen Vol. 1
Elizabeth II, H.M. Queen Vol. 1
Ensor, James Vol. 1
Erasmus, Desiderius Vol. 1
Etymology - Origin of the Word Fart 4-6
Family Guy Vol. 1
Fart, Colloquialism, Idiom, & Synonym 140-151
Fart, Etymology (Word Origin) 5-7
Fart, Foreign Language 152-154
Fart, Physiology 7-20
Fielding, Henry 58-59
Flaubert, Gustave 71-73
Foreign Languages 152-154
Fox, Charles James Vol. 1
Franklin, Benjamin Vol. 1
Fraser, George MacDonald 117-118

Freud, Sigmund Vol. 1
Gaddafi, Muammar Vol. 1
Gillray, James Vol. 1
Global Warming Vol. 1
Goethe, Johann Wolfgang Von 62-64
Goya, Francisco Vol. 1
Hadith, Islam Vol. 1
Hemingway, Ernest 105-106
Herodotus Vol. 1
Heywood, John 35-36
Hippocrates Vol. 1
Hitler, Adolf Vol. 1
Hugo, Victor 67-69
Hutchinson, Sir Robert Vol. 1
Huxley, Aldous 100-103
Idioms 140-151
Index 159-163
Introduction 1-3
Islam Hadith Vol. 1
Japanese Lithographs Edo Period Vol. 1
Jerome, Saint Vol. 1
Jonson, Ben 42-44
Johnson, Lyndon Baines Vol. 1
Johnson, Samuel 140
Josephus, Flavius Vol. 1
Joyce, James 97-99
Kant, Immanuel Vol. 1
Kuniyoshi, Utagawa Vol. 1
Lama, HH Dalai Vol. 1
Langland, William 30-31
Lawrence, D.H. 99-100
Lawrence (of Arabia), T.E. Vol. 1
Lear, Edward 69-70
Le Pétomane Vol. 1
Lincoln, Abraham Vol. 1
Lion King Vol. 1
Lord John Wilmot, Earl of Rochester 50-51
Ludlow, Henry Vol. 1
Luther, Martin Vol. 1
Mailer, Norman 114-115
Marchetta, Melina 133-134
Marketing & Advertising Vol. 1
Martialis, Marcus Valerius 25-26
Medieval Manuscripts Vol. 1
Metrocles Vol. 1
Michelangelo di Lodovico Buonarroti Simoni Vol. 1

Miller, Henry 104-105
Miller's Tale 180-182
Milton, John 22, 46-48
Montaigne, Michel de Vol. 1
Moore, Sir Thomas Vol. 1
Mozart, Wolfgang Amadeus Vol. 1
Movies Vol. 1
Mr. Methane Vol. 1
Nesbø, Jo 139
Newton, Richard Vol. 1
Oldfield, Paul Vol. 1
Ontario Ministry of Health Vol. 1
Patterson, James 128-130
Peasant's Fart 29-30
Petronius Vol. 1
Physiology – Digestion and the Fart 7-20
Piers Plowman 30-31
Plutarch Vol. 1
Preface VIII-IX
Prince Philip, HRH Vol. 1
Prophets, Bible Vol. 1
Pujol, Joseph Vol. 1
Pythagoras Vol. 1
Queen Elizabeth I, H.M Vol. 1
Queen Elizabeth II, H.M. Vol. 1
Rabelais, François 33-35
Reagan, Ronald Vol. 1
Rochester, Earl of, Lord John Wilmot 50-51
Roth, Philip 121-123
Rushdie, Salman 126-128
Rutebeuf 29-30
Saint Augustine Vol. 1
Saint Jerome Vol. 1
Salinger, J.D. 112-113
Seinfeld Vol. 1
Seneca Vol. 1
Shakespeare, William 36-40
Simpsons Vol. 1
Sir Richard Burton Vol. 1
Sir Winston Churchill Vol. 1
Sir Robert Hutchinson Vol. 1
Sir Thomas Moore Vol. 1
Sir Salman Rushdie 126-128
Sir John Suckling 45-46
South Park Vol. 1
Stalin, Josef Vol. 1

Stern, Howard 132-133
Stoutshanks, S. Vol. 1
Styron, William 115-116
Suckling, Sir John 45-46
Super Bowl Budweiser Commercial Vol. 1
Swift, Jonathon 51-54
Synonyms 140-151
Talmud, Babylonian Vol. 1
Tales of Gargantua and Pantagruel 33-35
Tibet, H.H. the 14th Dalai Lama Vol. 1
Toole, John Kennedy 119-120
Twain, Mark (Samuel Clemens) 73-93
Voltaire (François-Marie Arouet) 55-58
Von Goethe, Johann Wolfgang 62-64
Vonnegut, Jr., Kurt 113-114
Wagner, Richard Vol. 1
Warming, Global Vol. 1
Wells, William Vol. 1
Wenling, Chen Vol. 1
Whoopee Cushion Vol. 1
Wilmot, Lord John, Earl of Rochester 50-51
Wolfe, Thomas 106-108
Yoga Vol. 1
Zola, Émile 93-97

Made in the USA
Middletown, DE
11 October 2022